PSYCHOANALYTIC SUPERVISION

ALSO FROM NANCY McWILLIAMS

Psychoanalytic Case Formulation
Nancy McWilliams

Psychoanalytic Diagnosis: Understanding Personality
Structure in the Clinical Process, Second Edition
Nancy McWilliams

Psychoanalytic Psychotherapy: A Practitioner's Guide
Nancy McWilliams

Psychodynamic Diagnostic Manual, Second Edition (PDM-2)
Edited by Vittorio Lingiardi and Nancy McWilliams

Psychoanalytic

SUPERVISION

Nancy McWilliams

THE GUILFORD PRESS

New York   London

Printed in the United States of America

This book is printed on acid-free paper.

Last digit is print number: 9 8 7 6 5 4 3 2

The author has checked with sources believed to be reliable in the effort to provide information that is complete and generally in accord with her standards of practice that are accepted at the time of publication. However, in view of the possibility of human error or changes in behavioral, mental health, or medical sciences, neither the author, nor the editors and publisher, nor any other party who has been involved in the preparation or publication of this work warrants that the information contained herein is in every respect accurate or complete, and they are not responsible for any errors or omissions or the results obtained from the use of such information. Readers are encouraged to confirm the information contained in this book with other sources.

Library of Congress Cataloging-in-Publication Data

Names: McWilliams, Nancy, author.
Title: Psychoanalytic supervision / Nancy McWilliams.
Description: New York : The Guilford Press, 2021. | Includes
    bibliographical references and index.
Identifiers: LCCN 2021007546 | ISBN 9781462547999 (cloth)
Subjects: LCSH: Psychoanalysis--Study and teaching. |
    Psychotherapists—Supervision of. | Psychodynamic psychotherapy—Study
    and teaching.
Classification: LCC RC502 .M39 2021 | DDC 616.89/17076—dc23
LC record available at *https://lccn.loc.gov/2021007546*

For Michael Garrett
with love, admiration, and immeasurable gratitude

About the Author

Nancy McWilliams, PhD, ABPP, teaches in the Graduate School of Applied and Professional Psychology at Rutgers, The State University of New Jersey, and has a private practice in Lambertville, New Jersey. She is the author of *Psychoanalytic Diagnosis, Second Edition*; *Psychoanalytic Case Formulation*; and *Psychoanalytic Psychotherapy*; and coeditor of *Psychodynamic Diagnostic Manual, Second Edition* (PDM-2). She is a past president of the Society for Psychoanalysis and Psychoanalytic Psychology, Division 39 of the American Psychological Association (APA), and is on the editorial board of *Psychoanalytic Psychology*. A graduate of the National Psychological Association for Psychoanalysis, Dr. McWilliams is also affiliated with the Center for Psychotherapy and Psychoanalysis of New Jersey, and serves on the Board of Trustees of the Austen Riggs Center in Stockbridge, Massachusetts. She is a recipient of honors including the Gradiva Award from the National Association for the Advancement of Psychoanalysis; the Goethe Scholarship Award from the Section on Psychoanalytic and Psychodynamic Psychology of the Canadian Psychological Association; the Rosalee Weiss Award from the Division of Independent Practitioners of the APA; the Laughlin Distinguished Teacher Award from the American Society of Psychoanalytic Physicians; the Hans H. Strupp Award from the Appalachian Psychoanalytic Society; and the International, Leadership, and Scholarship Awards from APA Division 39. Dr. McWilliams is an honorary member of the American Psychoanalytic Association, the Moscow Psychoanalytic Society, the Institute for Psychoanalytic Psychotherapy of Turin, Italy, and the Warsaw Scientific Association for Psychodynamic Psychotherapy. Her writings have been translated into 20 languages.

Preface

This book organizes what I have learned about psychoanalytic supervision over a long career. Early in a professional life, it is hard to anticipate the shape of one's eventual contribution. Accidents of time and place foster unexpected specializations, research interests, and personal commitments. For me, it was pivotal that in the 1980s, shortly after the DSM had become a categorical, descriptive taxonomy whose clinical consequences I had begun to worry about, some of my students at the Rutgers Graduate School of Applied and Professional Psychology suggested that I write a primer on personality structure and its implications for treatment. My department chair, Stanley Messer, who knew that I enjoyed scholarly writing as well as teaching and practice, reinforced their message and kept me on task. I remain grateful, as these encouragements led to several decades of rewarding authorship. This book is probably my last textbook, but I have said that before. . . .

My clinical career started in 1973, when I worked in a local mental health center at the height of the community mental health movement. In those heady years, clinicians hoped to offer effective, life-changing psychotherapy to vast numbers of people. Psychological suffering was losing its stigma, the new antipsychotic medications were emptying the mental hospitals, and there were exciting new ways of conceptualizing how to help people. American insurance companies supported long-term treatments and deferred to therapists' judgments about what their patients needed. The United States was in an economically affluent period marked by idealism and the political will to improve the lives of even its most marginalized citizens.

It was an era (a brief one, in retrospect) when educational opportunities were plentiful, professionals had enough unscheduled time to get in-depth training on the job, and most young clinicians had considerable choice about supervisors. In addition to my two main mentors ("control analysts") at the National Psychological Association for Psychoanalysis, Arthur Robbins and the late Stanley Moldawsky, I sought supervision from psychoanalytically oriented psychologists (George Atwood, Bertram Cohen, Judith Klein, Milton Silva, and Duncan Walton), psychiatrists (Harmon Ephron and Iradj Siassi), and social workers (Judith Felton Logue and Herbert Strean). I got help with couple, family, and group therapy for adults, adolescents, and children. The late Sandra Leiblum introduced me to behavioral sex therapy; Monica McGoldrick taught me the basics of Bowenian family systems work; I was exposed to gestalt approaches and humanistic psychologies. I explored T-groups (the T is for "training"—an experiential learning model), transcendental meditation, and other enthusiasms of the day. I was able to absorb, and slowly integrate into my own supervisory approach, the styles of many talented teachers.

Looking back now after almost 50 years as a therapist and teacher myself, I can more clearly see the contours and themes of my vocation. They have consistently involved bringing the insights of the psychoanalytic community, and often the broader clinical community, to audiences outside professional in-groups—not only students of psychotherapy, but also academics, frontline service deliverers, community groups, and people of diverse backgrounds who are interested in the social construction of concepts such as individuality, mental health, psychopathology, and psychotherapy. Supervision and consultation are central ways of passing along psychoanalytic knowledge; they illuminate time-honored principles by foregrounding their application. At its best, supervision involves helping students to integrate the experiential legacy of clinical practice with what they have learned in academic programs. Throughout my career, I have enjoyed teaching roles in which I can foster such integrations, but now, in my mid-70s, I feel a particularly strong internal press to do so.

I can see in retrospect how accidents of my personal history contributed to this sense of mission. My mother died when I was 9 years old, leaving me with an idealization that had both negative and positive effects. In my 20s, psychoanalysis helped me with the negative repercussions. The positive effects included my internalizing the traditional maternal values of compassion and care that have infused my life and work. I inhabit a culture in which the "newest thing" is automatically preferred over older practices. The creation myth of the United States features breaking away from the mother country and starting something wholly new; Americans' favorite stories involve standing up against unimaginative or corrupt authorities. But in contrast to these familiar cultural tropes, my early loss left me with a deep appreciation of what has come before, what older generations offer us, and what can be lost in rushing toward the new.

This stance coexists with my professional history of trying to speak a modest kind of truth to power, probably largely out of an identification with my father's rock-ribbed honesty. In the current era, at least in Western societies, the interests of insurance companies, drug companies, political bodies, and some academics have drowned out the voices of those of us who know from experience what clinical practice is really like. At the same time, most of our professional organizations are more interested in recent discoveries than in time-tested understandings. Historical perspective, apprenticeship with seasoned teachers, and attention to artistic elements of therapeutic work have been devalued in favor of what is easy to measure.

I greatly value research on clinical topics (especially the practice- and person-oriented investigations that now counterbalance a previous narrow focus on trials of brief, manualized therapies for specific symptoms), and I have been dismayed when some psychoanalysts (including Freud) have minimized the importance of scientific investigation. I equally appreciate accumulated clinical wisdom (cf. Baltes, Glück, & Kunzmann, 2002; Baum-Baicker, 2018; Baum-Baicker & Sisti, 2012; Sternberg, 2003) and view psychoanalysis as one of many precious wisdom traditions whose insights are transmitted via stories, fables, metaphors, intuitive leaps, and subjective impressions. In a world increasingly divided into intellectual "silos," it is difficult for segregated communities to influence each other. A widening gulf between the worlds of practicing clinicians and those of academics (see Shedler, 2015; Shedler & Aftab, 2020) threatens a healthy equilibrium and creates cultures of misunderstanding and even contempt.

Here is just one example of the current imbalance. When practitioners submit a proposed workshop for continuing education credits, the American Psychological Association permits them to cite only scholarship published in the last 10 years, as if even exemplary work done more than a decade ago is worthless. (This strikes me as like saying, "Hasn't Herman Melville written anything lately?") Moreover, the "learning objectives" required in these applications must involve measurable achievements, a demand that has led to the peculiar result that teachers cannot use the term "learn" in the objectives they submit for continuing education credits.

This tilt toward a narrow empirical enthusiasm has always characterized American psychology, which is still trying to prove it is a "real" science. It is a bias that has sometimes had disturbing consequences (e.g., advice to not hug one's children, culturally insensitive IQ testing, the eugenics movement) that might have been avoided if enthusiasm for the newest ideas had been counterbalanced by the wisdom of communities with firsthand experience, especially those with comparatively less privilege and power than the psychologists promulgating the newest intellectual fad.

In the contemporary academic environment, it is easy to forget that the insights of dedicated clinicians (e.g., Bleuler on psychotic experience, Winnicott on play) can be more useful to therapists than the latest contribution from the psych lab. Supervision is an area in which clinical experience and accumulated clinical knowledge are particularly critical. Like therapy, supervision is an art. It should be informed by science, but it is not equivalent to science. It should indeed be "evidence based." But in my view, that evidence should include not only randomized controlled trials, but also the accrued reflections of clinicians with years of seasoning. It is well known that subjective reports are suspect, that memory is unreliable, and that one compelling anecdote does not establish a principle. It is less appreciated that objective data can be misinterpreted, compromised, or misapplied as well. I try in this book to offer supervisors both empirical findings and the wisdom of many decades of communal experience in the arts of mentoring and being mentored.

Until fairly recently, people learned to supervise mostly by trial and error. They depended, as I did, on their internalizations of their supervisors, feedback from their supervisees, and clinical evidence that clients were improving in response to a mentor's suggestion. In recent years, the American Psychological Association, hoping to prepare psychologists for supervisory roles in integrated health care systems, has asked graduate programs in clinical psychology to include courses on supervision in their curricula. Psychiatric organizations, similarly concerned that medical residents prepare adequately for the supervisory roles they will fill in hospital hierarchies, are making parallel recommendations. This development is long overdue.

As such courses are created, there has been an increase both in the empirical study of supervision and in commentaries by seasoned mentors on the supervisory process. New instruments for studying supervision are appearing, and new systematic approaches are being developed. It seems a good time for an overview and integration of psychoanalytic reflections on the topic. In contrast to the current literature that emphasizes skills training—a worthy goal that has the advantage of being easy to conceptualize, research, and teach—in this book I focus more on the *gestalt* of supervision and its role in promoting maturation, confidence, and a sense of agency in the therapist. As in my books on diagnosis, case formulation, and psychotherapy, I am trying to keep accumulated clinical experience alive and in view alongside what research can teach us.

This emphasis on received wisdom and a respect for accumulated clinical experience may be more typical of programs in educational and developmental psychology, counseling, social work, and pastoral care than programs in contemporary clinical psychology and psychiatry. And, from my perspective, the emphasis on wisdom and clinical experience is more reflective of clinical realities. These include the empirically demonstrated fact that there are different ways to treat mental health problems effectively, the finding that even disorders meeting the same DSM criteria have different meanings in different people and thus require different relational skills (see, e.g., Norcross & Wampold, 2019), and the commonsense notion that supervisory styles must be integrated into one's authentic personality.

This book is intended for mental health professionals of all disciplines and backgrounds. Even though it is fundamentally psychoanalytic, I am hoping it will be of value to readers without prior exposure to psychodynamic theories or therapies. I have tried to avoid jargon and to make examples relevant to a broad range of clinical situations. I hope that it will be useful to readers of diverse theoretical orientations and at all levels of the supervisory process, from seasoned professionals, who are usually appreciative of a fresh perspective on how to help newer colleagues, to beginning clinicians digesting their first experience of being supervised. I have enjoyed putting these ideas together. I hope you enjoy reading them.

Acknowledgments

My primary debt is to Malin Fors, who originally urged me to write this book. She has conferred with me throughout the process, both from the perspective of having consulted with me on her cases for more than a decade, and from the perspective of her own many years as a mentor to therapists of widely divergent backgrounds who work in widely varying situations. Malin has made numerous specific recommendations that I have implemented; for example, she suggested that I include ideas about dealing with "disastrous" supervisees and counseling them out of the field—not my primary interest, but a critical issue that belongs in a book on this topic.

My second debt is to all the supervisors mentioned earlier whose voices now speak through me. I argue in this book that becoming a good supervisor is much more about one's identifications than about what one masters cognitively, and my own internalizations of former supervisors run deep. I want to note especially the influence of Arthur Robbins, to whom I dedicated a previous text, and to George Atwood, whose phenomenological approach to making sense of clinical material has had an enduring effect on how I think clinically. My belief that getting consultation from valued colleagues should be a lifelong process also comes from personal experience. When I run into clinical challenges, I consult with Kerry Gordon or Joyce Slochower, friends who are candid with their criticisms and consoling with their loving support.

I thank Judy Ann Kaplan for generously sharing a personal speech on the topic of supervision and for offering me several years of syllabi for her course at the National Psychological Association for Psychoanalysis. Brian Chu and Karen Skean, my colleagues at the Graduate School of Applied and Professional Psychology at Rutgers University, were similarly generous with syllabi and bibliographies on supervision from a range of theoretical perspectives. I am indebted to Hanne Strømme and Siri Gullestad and their colleagues at the Nordic Psychotherapy Training Study at the University of Oslo, who have generously shared their research findings and their reflections on them. Robert Feinstein at Dell Medical School in Austin, Texas, enlightened me about his interesting approach to supervising medical residents. On several occasions I have co-supervised with Jonathan Shedler, or witnessed his consultations with others; these experiences have expanded my own supervisory style.

Kerry Gordon read several sections of the manuscript with his usual sensitivity; I particularly appreciate his suggestion of the concept of "vital signs" for the material in Chapter 3. I thank Lynne Harkless, Otto Kernberg, Babak Rashanaei-Moghaddam, Helene Schwartzbach, Dhwani Shah, Neil Skolnick, and Shawn Sobkowski for sharing their observations about the special challenges of supervision in psychoanalytic institutes and members of my consultation and supervision groups for giving me feedback on group supervision. I appreciate also the thoughtful last-minute critiques of Chapters 8 and 9 from Drew Mendelson and Tanya Llewellyn.

I am grateful to organizations that have asked me to speak on supervision, including the Center for Psychotherapy and Psychoanalysis of New Jersey, the California Psychological Association, Richmond Area Multi-Services in San Francisco, and counseling centers at the University of San Diego, the University of California at Los Angeles, Villanova University, and Seton Hall University. Jan-Martin Berge organized a program about professional growth in Oslo, Norway, that proved highly stimulating, as was a subsequent presentation that Ida Bernhardt and Inger Selvaag organized at the Oslo University counseling services.

Every clinician I have supervised or consulted with has taught me something valuable, whether I talked with that colleague in a one-time consult or repeatedly over many years. I have been especially stimulated by the therapists in my private consulting groups and in my weekly class at Rutgers. A special shout-out to my Chinese colleagues, Wu Chunyan (Amy Wu) and Wang Shaoyu, for our regular conversations about supervision. I am grateful to the impressive therapists in Norway's prison system for insights I have gleaned from our ongoing consultations. To the many practitioners brave enough to expose their work to me at conferences and workshops, I express my thanks.

This is the fourth book I have worked on with Kitty Moore, my editor at The Guilford Press. Her reaching out to me 30 years ago after a talk I had given on dissociative psychology, to inquire whether I had any book plans, ushered in a new era in my professional life and gave me a trusted friend and confidante. Kitty got behind *Psychoanalytic Diagnosis* when it was only a gleam in my eye, before I had any reputation as a writer or scholar. She gave me useful advice on organization, helped me sharpen up core ideas, shepherded me through details of manuscript preparation, and promoted the book to her colleagues at Guilford. She has midwifed this one with her usual thoroughness and enthusiasm, for which I am grateful.

Finally, and most vitally, I have learned, and continue to learn, a prodigious amount from Michael Garrett, to whom this book is dedicated. I was lucky to meet Michael, years after we had both lost devoted spouses, and to marry him late in life. As a consultant to therapists throughout the world who are trying to help people with psychosis, and as a supervisor of psychiatric residents in a public hospital setting, working to improve the lives of the most devastated patients among the urban poor, Michael has managed to bring knowledge, skill, and hope to generations of practitioners. He consults on my cases when I ask for his help (a frequent occurrence) and has made many useful editorial suggestions for this manuscript. But his influence on my understanding of supervision goes much further than such advice. It is not often that one gets to witness a master supervisor up close, but I have had that privilege with Michael, and I am a better mentor because of it. Most consequentially for this book, his love, emotional support, and empathic resonance, deriving from the remarkable parallels in our respective commitments to our professional missions, keep me nourished and excited about our work.

Contents

Introduction

C. E. Watkins, Jr., a preeminent scholar on psychoanalytic and humanistic mentorship, offers a definition of psychoanalytic supervision from Bernard and Goodyear (2009, p. 7):

> An educational method or intervention where a more knowledgeable, experienced, and senior member of the psychoanalytic profession enters into a relationship with a less knowledgeable, less experienced, junior member . . . to enhance the professional functioning of that junior member's practice and conceptual skills; that professional relationship typically is evaluative and hierarchical, extends over time, and involves monitoring of quality and quality control. (quoted in Watkins, 2011, p. 403)

In accordance with this description, I have oriented these ideas toward all practitioners whose clinical work is grounded in psychodynamic understanding. Although I devote a portion of this work (Chapter 7) to supervision in psychoanalytic institutes, I do not intend the book to be read exclusively, or even predominantly, by analysts. In fact, I am hoping that supervisors of other perspectives will find it applicable to their work, as I suspect that—just as effective therapy correlates with relational factors more than treatment "brand"—the quality of any supervision is independent of the theoretical orientation of the supervisor.

LEARNING FROM PAST ACCOMPLISHMENTS AND MISTAKES

This hope for relevance to supervisors of diverse backgrounds is consistent with the fact that the history of psychoanalytic supervision is the history of clinical supervision itself. Because the Freudian project offered the first systematic approach to psychotherapy and thus the first literature on how to train people to do it, there is a great deal of general clinical value in that body of work. At the same time, the analytic literature has been guilty of numerous omissions, biases, and missteps; I discuss some of those failings in pertinent areas of this book. It would be a shame for contemporary practitioners to repeat historical errors in supervision that the analytic community once ignorantly committed and has come to regret.

One mistake many psychoanalysts have made involves framing supervision as indoctrination into a particular technical approach (e.g., teaching an idealized version of interpretation or positing unbreakable rules of therapeutic engagement) rather than construing their mentorship as enabling supervisees to develop a style of work that suits both themselves and their patients. I was once critiqued by a senior analyst for having helped a patient greatly, but not in a properly orthodox way. I viewed this as the inverse of the joke, "The operation was successful, but the patient died." In my case, the operation was judged unsuccessful despite the fact that the patient flourished. That experience left me dubious about idealizing reified methods at the expense of the individuality of the patient and at the expense of the outcome that the rules had been invented to reach.

Currently, there are echoes of this reifying tendency in psychologists' enthusiasm for skills-training models. This text draws from some of that focused work in its emphasis on teaching supervisees how to establish with patients an alliance built on a mutual understanding of treatment goals, of how psychodynamic therapies work, and about what to expect the clinician's and patient's respective roles to be in the clinical process. Although training in specific skills and in "deliberate practice" can be valuable, I think it is at the same time important not to reduce supervision to the teaching of particular procedures and to keep in mind a larger vision of professional development (cf. Ladany, 2007). That bigger picture is what this book is about.

There are several recent books on general clinical supervision that are applicable to psychoanalytic work (e.g., Bernard & Goodyear, 2018; Falender & Shafranske, 2016; Watkins & Milne, 2014), as well as a number specifically devoted to psychodynamic supervision (e.g., Szecsödy,

2013). Classic psychoanalytic writings on supervision, in chronological order, include texts by Ekstein and Wallerstein (1958/1971), Wallerstein (1981), Benedek and Fleming (1983), Caligor, Bromberg, and Meltzer (1984), Dewald (1987), Jacobs, David, and Meyer (1995), and Frawley-O'Dea and Sarnat (2001). Some good edited collections of papers on the topic have been offered by Martindale, Mörner, Cid Rodriguez, and Vidit (1997), Rock (1997), Weiner, Mizen, and Duckham (2003), Petts and Shapley (2007), and Hess, Hess, and Hess (2008). More recently, we have had important contributions from Joan Sarnat (2015) and Jill Savege Scharff (2018). Although these various writers have represented different theoretical orientations and evolving visions of the psychoanalytic process, their views are not significantly at odds with one another. This fact has made my own integrative approach easier to accomplish than it would have been if the field were awash in controversy.

The information in this book is compatible with much of what these authors have had to say. (Given the degree to which we both eschew binaries and emphasize emotional safety, readers will probably find my own sensibility most comparable to that of Joan Sarnat.) The material in this book differs somewhat from those of my predecessors, however; it covers some ground that I have not seen explored as thoroughly as it might be, including a focus on the ways analytic clinicians evaluate progress, the benefits of group supervision and consultation, and the effects of institute dynamics on supervisors and supervisees. It also contains some direct advice to supervisees.

ORGANIZATION

Supervision involves a somewhat different skill set than that required in practicing psychotherapy, and certainly different challenges and complications, as implied by the quality-control part of Watkins's (2011) definition. It requires even more maturity, comfort in authority, and nuanced judgment than clinical work does. There are many ways of organizing the complex material relevant to such maturation. I have chosen to go roughly from the general and historical to the specific and contemporary. In Chapter 1, I discuss the goals and processes involved in psychoanalytic supervision, framing it as an intimate kind of education. I emphasize offering support, promoting honesty, providing information, teaching skills, nurturing an ethical sensibility, socializing colleagues into a psychoanalytic ethos, and preventing burnout. Chapter 2 covers the history of psychoanalytic supervision, from Freud's ideas through contemporary relational work on the supervisory alliance. There I address two recurrent tensions in the field: whether to teach or to treat and whether to impart specific techniques or foster general professional maturity.

Because the psychodynamic tradition has framed desirable clinical outcomes as involving much more than the alleviation of manifest symptoms, I have devoted Chapter 3 to an explication of what constitutes progress in a psychodynamic therapy. To supervise effectively, one must have a concept of what comprises psychological wellness, that is, what the supervisee and the client are working *toward*. I suggest 10 "vital signs" of therapeutic progress: greater attachment security; improved self- and object constancy; increased sense of agency; movement toward more realistic and reliable self-esteem; greater resilience and affect regulation; more ability to reflect on the self and mentalize others; increased comfort in both communality and individuality; a more robust sense of vitality; the development of improved capacities for acceptance, forgiveness, and gratitude; and finally, the overarching capacities to love, work, and play.

Chapter 4 delves into individual supervision in some depth, including the supervisory contract, the formulation of realistic treatment goals, and the promotion of frankness in the supervisory dyad. I mention some resistances to learning, recommend ways of playing with alternative solutions to clinical problems, introduce some general ethical concerns, and emphasize the value of the supervisee's own psychotherapy. The chapter closes with some reflections on the gratifications of supervision. In Chapter 5, I explore group supervision and consultation, including considerable material about my own work within this model. I address some resistances and complications and conclude with observations about the advantages of supervisory work with groups of therapists and counselors.

Given the critical role of supervisors in monitoring patient care and in protecting the public from inadequate or destructive clinicians, I have devoted an entire chapter to supervisors' ethical obligations. Chapter 6 offers certain orienting premises, including what patients have the right to know, and then explores ethical dilemmas involving the best interests of the client and the community, respectively. The chapter contains extensive vignettes illustrating the complexity of ethical challenges and concludes with attention to evaluation procedures and gatekeeping responsibilities.

Issues of training in psychoanalytic institutes have been deeply fraught, both historically and in the present. Consequently, I decided to include a chapter devoted entirely to the mentoring of institute candidates. Chapter 7 reviews both the satisfactions and unique challenges of that work. Among the latter are regressive dynamics, issues of psychoanalytic identity, problematic consequences of idealization and devaluation, and splitting. I focus on numerous vexed issues, including systemic pressures that sometimes operate to the disadvantage of both supervisees and patients. I make specific recommendations for avoiding some of the worst pitfalls that can complicate supervision in the hothouse cultures of psychoanalytic training.

Just as every patient (and every therapist–patient dyad) is unique, so too is every combination of supervisor and supervisee. Nonetheless, in Chapter 8, I generalize about certain psychological tendencies that can characterize either party in the supervisory relationship. Specifically, I discuss the consequences of dynamics involved in depressive and masochistic, paranoid, schizoid, hysterical, obsessive–compulsive, posttraumatic, narcissistic, and psychopathic psychologies, and talk about some ways of dealing with those tendencies. I then address other areas of individual difference as they may affect supervision and consultation, including (but not limited to) gender, sexuality, race and ethnicity, class, culture, religious and spiritual background and affinities, political orientation, oppression, and privilege generally.

Chapter 9 differs from the tone of scholarly overview in the preceding chapters. In it, I take an explicit advisory role, speaking directly to supervisees about how to get the most out of their experiences of clinical training. I suggest a vision of what supervision at its best can do for one's professional and personal growth, and I comment on the cognitive and emotional demands of clinical work for which therapists' academic training may not have prepared them. I frame the goals of supervision in terms of (1) developing a guiding internal supervisory voice and (2) learning when and how to seek consultation throughout one's career. I try to help supervisees to mentalize their supervisors, to deal with supervisory situations that are difficult or even damaging, and to find the courage to look at their own contributions to any problems with patients and/or mentors.

ETHICAL CONSIDERATIONS AND TERMINOLOGY

As in my previous writing, I draw liberally on my own experience to illustrate the material I cover. All vignettes about students, colleagues, consultees, supervisees, and patients have either been approved by the people in question or disguised in conformance with contemporary professional standards. As all psychoanalytic writers know, it is hard to retain the integrity of a clinical description while distorting identifying features of the people involved. I hope I have kept undamaged the essential truths in the anecdotes I include.

With respect to terminology, I use the term "supervision" generically but sometimes differentiate it from consultation. I understand consultation to be voluntary on the part of the learner, that is, not required by a training program or third party. In consultations, the supervisor has no legal obligation to others to evaluate the colleague. I sometimes use the broader terms "mentor," "mentee," and "mentorship" to refer to both supervision and consultation; when I use the term "trainee," it specifically applies to students in graduate or postgraduate training programs. As in my other books, I do not typically distinguish between "psychoanalytic" and "psychodynamic," I use "patient" and "client" synonymously, and I refer to mental health professionals interchangeably as "therapists," "clinicians," "counselors," and "practitioners."

Chapter One

■ ■ ■ ■

Overview of
Psychoanalytic Supervision

One can easily make the case that good supervision is simply good supervision, irrespective of the theoretical orientation of the supervisor, therapist, or clinical setting. In many respects, I subscribe to this view, and in fact much of what I say in this book is applicable to any kind of supervision. But there are some distinctive elements of psychoanalytic clinical wisdom, less emphasized in other approaches, that I highlight here. This chapter covers areas relevant to therapists' clinical maturation, with specific attention to some ways that conscientious supervisors can facilitate their less experienced colleagues' personal and professional growth.

Supervision of clinical work is best located under the heading of education, one of the three professions (along with healing and governing) that Freud (1937) famously depicted as intrinsically "impossible." Psychoanalytic supervision may be uniquely and even perversely impossible, as it attempts an ambitious, intimate, emotional education that goes far beyond the teaching of protocols. Analysts have always appreciated the fact that while people are ingesting information, they may learn from a teacher's attitude, tone, and behavior some lessons that are deeper than what is overtly and consciously taken in.

Psychoanalytic therapists are sensitive to subtle and unstated emotional valences. We pay particular attention to the gestalt of supervisory

7

activities. As every parent should know, when a child is harshly shamed, even when the content of the caregiver's criticism is apt, the main lessons the child is likely to learn include that harsh shaming is okay, the self is contemptible, and authorities should be feared. In parallel, as I suggested in the Introduction, although contemporary graduate training tends to emphasize the transmission of specific, preferably measurable clinical skills, the feelings that surround this process can be much more important than the skills themselves. Ideally, supervision offers plentiful opportunities to identify with mentors who exemplify a therapeutic attitude. For this reason, in the following account of educative tasks facing psychodynamic supervisors, I begin with the recommended emotional tone of psychoanalytic supervision.

PROVIDING PSYCHOLOGICAL SUPPORT

From their mentors, therapists need to learn how to weather storms of negative feeling coming directly at them from miserable people, how to keep their self-esteem when being relentlessly devalued, how to recognize and deal with the grain of truth in patients' complaints about them, how to handle their traumatic internal responses to searing accounts of trauma, how to bear ugly and personally alien feelings in themselves, how to tolerate uncertainty, how to set boundaries with people who feel wounded by reasonable limits, how to maintain an unnatural level of secret keeping, how to find hope when clients fill the office with their despair, how to manage anxieties that a patient may die by suicide, and other emotionally taxing lessons.

Some of these areas are particularly demanding for clinicians who are just starting to work psychodynamically. An ambitious review of the clinical literature by Blagys and Hilsenroth (2000) revealed that what practicing therapists consider definitional of dynamic treatment includes attention to the transference (i.e., we "work in the transference," "interpret the negative transference," "tolerate an intense transference," or "accept a self-object transference," and so on). Psychodynamic clinicians must become comfortable exploring the immediate emotional complexities, including the less conscious negative aspects, of the therapeutic relationship. The challenge of helping patients to be honest with themselves in the here and now about disowned, minimized, or rationalized feelings toward us requires us to be similarly honest about our own subjective world. I have found that it is hard for most new therapists to make the critical shift from what is more natural to them—that is, trying to demonstrate to patients their superiority to their earlier caregivers—to the less natural attitude of welcoming of their client's experiences that they are just as bad.

In addition, therapists may need to *unlearn* mindsets that have previously been adaptive professionally or personally. These may include a tendency toward people pleasing, or an inclination toward advice giving, or a self-protective avoidance of others' accurate perceptions of one's limitations and failings, or a tendency to respond automatically to a person's problem by describing how one resolved a comparable problem of one's own, or a proclivity to fall too easily into the stance of "the one who knows." The last kind of unlearning may be particularly challenging for medically trained therapists, who for prior professional responsibilities have had to take to heart the message "You're the doctor. You're in charge!" How to come to a sense of confidence that one is an expert in supporting the *process* of therapy, while not claiming a superior position about the *content* of any patient's mental life, is a complicated personal evolution.

Finally, professionals learning how to do psychoanalytic therapy need to integrate being authentically themselves with being in a role that invites patients to make them into whoever the patient currently needs to see them as being. Anyone who has been through the process of putting together the combination of staying in role while not "playing" a role knows that achieving that integration takes years, minimally involving the 10,000 hours of practice required by musicians for excellence (Ericsson, Krampe, & Tesch-Römer, 1993) that Malcolm Gladwell (2011) famously popularized as a general norm. During that time, exposure to exemplars of how to inhabit a therapeutic role is critical. Even for seasoned analysts, being the target of intense transferences is never a walk in the park. But because it does get easier over time, mentors can forget how hard it was for them in their early years to remain fully themselves, both internally and with respect to how they carried out their therapeutic role, in the face of a patient's insistent feeling that the clinician is "really" someone else. In that process of maintaining authenticity while remaining in role, alongside all the cognitive areas they need to master, supervisees need respect, sympathy, and what Benjamin (2017) has elegantly theorized as *recognition*; that is, the supervisor's capacity to identify with each supervisee, to appreciate the person's individuality, to make him or her feel seen and accepted.

Perhaps the central challenge for psychoanalytic supervisors involves the balance between critical feedback and emotional support. Naturally, the pendulum is heavier on the supportive side when students are just beginning their immersion in psychoanalytic work and changes over time as they become more comfortable in the role of therapist. A sensitive supervisor takes into consideration the supervisee's level of professional development and is mindful of the fact that to continue to be a cheerleader once the newer colleague is more seasoned would be infantilizing.

That said, let me note that the supervisor's job is to help supervisees keep learning despite the fact that *any* learning—but especially the new knowledge one has to absorb as a therapist—is hard on one's self-esteem. Being confronted with what we did not already know, or what we were wrong about, is painful. Tact, warmth, and timeliness in dosing the information a supervisee needs to know come naturally to some supervisors, while others describe ongoing struggles to remind themselves that the individuals they mentor, while often impressively smart and competent, are still vulnerable to sudden, severe injury to their self-esteem (see Gill, 1999).

I remember, for example, a graduate student who confessed to me, "My whole life attests to the fact that I'm pretty smart, but this devaluing patient has made me feel like the village idiot." A seasoned colleague sought supervision with me because, for the first time, she found herself full of fantasies of murdering a relentlessly provocative patient. Another supervisee told me that for the first time in years he was having traumatic dreams that were clearly related to a patient's treating him the way a childhood abuser had behaved. I remember telling one of my own supervisors, "I can't get this patient to see that his transference *is* a transference! He thinks I'm exactly like his hateful mother. How can I get him to see that I'm trying to help him?" (Answer: That won't happen for a while, and meanwhile, it looks like you're going to have to live with feeling misunderstood.) It would be hard to overstate the importance of conveying to supervisees that one appreciates the chronic assaults on one's self-esteem that come with the territory of being in the role of both therapist and student.

PROMOTING HONEST ENGAGEMENT AND GOOD USE OF SUPERVISION

Frank revelations of everything we think and feel in a relationship is not part of ordinary social discourse. In fact, full disclosure is a more or less foolproof way to lose the good will of one's friends and relatives. In a psychoanalytic treatment, however, it is the "basic rule," and one that patients find very hard to follow (perceptively, some analysts have noted that the capacity to engage in completely "free" association is not usually psychologically possible until the end of a psychoanalytic treatment). Just as it is difficult for patients to accept the invitation to say everything that comes to mind about their thoughts, feelings, and behaviors, it is hard for clinicians to represent their work to supervisors with complete candor. Even supervision via video or audio recordings offers possibilities for avoiding complete self-exposure; in any supervisory hour, therapists can choose which part of the recording they will play, or they can fail to mention what happened at the start and the end of the session when the recording devices were off. Especially when a supervisor is legally or institutionally responsible for evaluating the clinician's work, complete disclosure is frightening to clinicians, particularly to those in the early phases of their careers, who worry that they are making one mistake after another.

Some fortunate beginning therapists have studied music, acting, or the visual arts. They generally have become more accepting of certain realities: that there are different ways to approach a task, that one never attains some fantasied ideal of perfection, that most clinical decisions are trade-offs rather than a matter of doing the right thing versus the wrong one, that one needs critical feedback throughout one's professional life, and that professional criticism does not equate with personal attack. Clinicians with a background in the arts are already familiar with integrating technique into their authentic self and with working flexibly, as it suits their personalities, from general principles. But most new therapists lack that experience. Those with mainly academic backgrounds are accustomed to striving for A's on tests and papers, a pursuit that reinforces irrational perfectionism and the illusion that there is a "right answer" (see Arkowitz, 2001). As a result, they tend to feel personally inadequate when a supervisor points out that they could have done something different in a session.

In addition, there is both anecdotal and empirical evidence that many therapists have depressively organized personalities (see Hyde, 2009; McWilliams, 2004). They are attracted to the role of helper because their self-esteem is supported (and their negative self-states are counteracted) by doing good in the world. They have big hearts. They also tend toward guilt, are self-critical, and easily internalize negative evaluations. When a client is doing well in treatment, they credit the client's talent and hard work; when a client is doing badly, they feel it must be their own fault. Hence, because of the effects of both the supervisory situation itself and the typical personal dispositions of therapists, it would be a mistake for a supervisor to underestimate how easily any clinician can feel shamefully exposed and reprimanded. Only the most narcissistic or psychopathic supervisees—thankfully rare in our profession—lack an inner voice channeling every past critic of their deficiencies.

Sensitive supervisors develop a style of communication that acknowledges the positive features of a clinician's work while suggesting something else the person could have done that may have had a better result. The usual psychological advice to offer good feedback before bad applies particularly to supervision. Here are some examples of how a tactful supervisor might implement this rule of thumb:

- "It sounds like your patient has gotten more relaxed and open with you despite her problems with trust. That is no small thing; it shows how well you've worked with her. But at the same time, I find myself wondering if both of you are avoiding areas where her distrust is still active, and seeking safety in a kind of tacit agreement that her tendency toward paranoia is completely behind her."

- "I get why you felt you had to let the session run over. I think I would have done the same thing given how much emotional pressure the client put on you to give him a little extra time. But I suspect that your decision to extend the time may cause problems in the long run, as it might reinforce his apparent feeling that because he's suffered a lot, he's entitled to have the rules modified on his behalf. You may have inadvertently created problems for yourself."

- "That was brilliant! Do you think she took it in, or is it just you and I who can see how right you were?"

No matter how sensitive and supportive we are in our supervisory role, however, we cannot prevent some shame and pain in people we are trying to mentor. Negative responses to supervision are inevitable: Even the simple experience of learning something that one did not already know involves a small narcissistic injury. Attunement to how supervisees respond to one's feedback, especially the negative side of their feeling, is a vital part of the psychoanalytic supervisory process. Just as the expression of anger or hurt by a patient toward a therapist opens clinical work to deeper insights, the admission of negative reactions by supervisees toward supervisors can facilitate and deepen their work together.

Usually, this freedom to disagree or confess a negative reaction takes a long time to develop, especially with supervisees whose work is under evaluation by their program, but it is a valuable goal for supervisors to keep in mind. When emotion is not processed, cognitive mastery can be incomplete and fragile (see Bucci & Maski, 2007; Castonguay & Hill, 2007; Vivona, 2013). Sometimes, supervisees rightly feel it would be unwise to admit to some of their criticisms of a mentor, and often they learn a lot anyway (Strømme, 2014; Strømme & Gullestad, 2012), but ideally a supervisor who can tolerate their critical questions and negative responses can give them a more deeply authentic experience.

Occasionally, a supervisor needs to address a defense that the super-visee regularly uses to protect against narcissistic injury. Dealing with defenses with a supervisee is not very different from doing so with a patient: one needs timing, tact, and a readiness to show how the defensive reaction is getting in the way of learning and growth. A common defense in supervision, for example, is preemptive self-attack. Even though most therapists may be inclined toward self-criticism, some of them go fur-ther: They begin almost every supervisory session with a confession of sins. The hour feels like a litany of "I think I screwed up here, I think I screwed up there. . . . " The supervisor soon gets the sense that there is a self-protective calculation involved: "If I attack myself first, the inevi-table attack of the supervisor won't feel so bad. And if I haven't screwed up, the supervisor will reassure me, and that will feel good."

When such transference-based expectations interfere with uncom-plicated learning, it may be useful for supervisors to name them and to help the less experienced colleague distinguish the current situation from earlier experiences of being shamed and disparaged. Once a defen-sive pattern of this sort has become visible to both supervisor and clini-cian, the two parties can note its regular occurrence, and the mentor can express good-humored empathy for the phenomenon (most supervisors probably did this themselves in their early years as practitioners). Then the supervisor can point out that although the knee-jerk self-attacks seem to do no harm, they do consume a certain amount of time and energy that could be better spent simply saying what happened in a ses-sion and getting the supervisor's ideas about the clinical process.

Defensiveness can sometimes characterize supervisors as well, requiring some self-analysis and possibly consultation with colleagues. Welcoming of negative reactions is a distinguishing feature of psycho-analytic work. In my personal journey learning to be a therapist, noth-ing went further in making me feel like an adult professional than hav-ing my communications, especially my criticisms, taken seriously and without defensiveness by supervisors. Because my father was something of a know-it-all, and I consequently expected authorities to be defensive, I remember numerous instances of being surprised and relieved by supervisory responses, such as a curiosity to learn more about my point of view, a willingness to rethink an opinion, or apologies for misunderstanding. Such experiences taught me a lot about the nature of benevolently authoritative, as opposed to authoritarian, mentoring.

Inviting and empowering supervisees to bring up anything that is bothering them is central to collaborative supervisory work. Speaking truth to one's mentors should contribute to the supervisee's helping patients do the same. In my role as a facilitator of groups of advanced clinical graduate students, there have been numerous times when a beginning therapist became brave enough to criticize something I said or did. I mention some experiences of this sort in Chapter 5. When group members see that the confrontation evokes my interest and serious self-scrutiny rather than the retaliation they fear, the group dynamic moves to a deeper, safer level. Via such experiences, members may get progressively more comfortable with the inevitable confrontations they will face from patients.

PROVIDING INFORMATION

Supervisees need help in many areas in which supervisors have come to know more than they do. Domains in which they may simply need more knowledge include such practical matters as the details of the policies of the clinical setting where they work, information on local laws and ethics relevant to treatment, billing and record-keeping procedures, third-party payer requirements, information about self-help resources such as twelve-step programs, and education about what they can expect and should do when an attorney contacts them. They can be informed about useful articles and books, research germane to their clinical population, upcoming conferences, and relevant podcasts. They can be told about organizations that support what they do and that provide access to findings that can help them make good clinical judgments.

They can profit as well from information about general topics relevant to treatment, including both clinical and empirical literatures in areas like personality differences, maturational processes, neuroscience, affect, trauma, addiction, and attachment. They need to be exposed to different models of treatments within and outside the psychodynamic arena so that they have a good basis for making referrals beyond their own sphere of competence. A minimal knowledge of common medications for psychological conditions is valuable, as is information on well-regarded local psychiatrists and other health professionals. Awareness of social programs that can help patients (i.e., the kind of expertise that social workers typically possess) can come in very handy for supervisees, especially for those treating patients with complex psychopathology who need external as well as internal changes in their lives. In addition, they may benefit from knowing a bit about laws affecting insurance corporations and from related tips on how to deal with threats from such companies to the continuity of treatment.

It is clinically useful to have some knowledge of different cultures, minority groups, job-related identity groups, and other identifiable populations not defined by a *disorder* (e.g., twins, adoptees, transgender individuals, people who were treated as a substitute for a sibling who died, bereaved children, children of divorce, children of addicts, survivors of cults, people with physical difficulties and chronic illnesses, the very old, and so on). Any supervisor who has practiced for a few years will have accumulated an impressive range of knowledge in such areas that may be completely new information to a less seasoned therapist.

Finally, it is currently a regrettable reality that psychodynamically oriented supervisees need a knowledge of data to cite when responding to misunderstandings and devaluations of psychoanalytic scholarship and practice. In the United States, except for therapists in some urban centers, knowing the research literature well enough to refute widespread fallacies about psychoanalysis (e.g., that there is no "evidence base" for it, or that no reputable professional does analytic treatment anymore, or that everything psychodynamic has been empirically discredited) is a requirement these days for surviving as a psychodynamic practitioner. There is an upside, however, to the burden of having to correct misguided colleagues: When others find out (through frequent, patient, nondefensive responses to their dismissive statements) that the psychoanalytic tradition is not the empirical wasteland that some ignorant professor told them it was, they are often interested in learning psychodynamic concepts that are clinically valuable.

Recently (late March 2020), on an active international listserv for psychoanalytic researchers on which I lurk, participating scientists agreed upon a list of the best empirical investigations of psychodynamic therapy, most of which are ambitious meta-analyses. The following studies comprised their top recommendations: Abbass, Rabung, Leichsenring, Refseth, and Midgely (2013); Abbass et al. (2014); Barlow, Bennett, Midgley, Larkin, and Wei (2015); Driessen et al. (2015);

Hayes, Gelso, Goldberg, and Kivlighan (2018); Høglend et al. (2006); Keefe, McCarthy, Dinger, Zilcha-Mano, and Barber (2014); Leichsenring, Luyten, Hilsenroth, Abbass, and Barber (2015); Shedler (2010); Steinert, Munder, Rabung, Hoyer, and Leichsenring (2017); and Westen (1998). I include them here for the benefit of any supervisors who are in the familiar situation of being asked by supervisees for scientific evidence supporting the psychoanalytic therapies. Those who express such concerns can be directed also to the extensive empirical literature on issues like attachment, personality, development, defensive processes, and neuroscience, all of which have significant implications for clinical practice.

TEACHING SKILLS

Psychoanalytic practice embodies a particular sensibility, or a set of attitudes and values that in themselves create a potentially therapeutic atmosphere (Brenner & Khan, 2013; Buechler, 2004; McWilliams, 2004; Schafer, 1983; Thompson, 2004). Psychodynamic supervisors need to teach or facilitate the techniques and competencies reflecting the sensibility that practitioners have developed over time through clinical trial and error as well as research. Different writers have parsed these skills differently (e.g., Abbass, 2004; Beitman & Yue, 2004; De Masi, 2019; Plakun, Sudak, & Goldberg, 2009; Rousmaniere, 2016; Sarnat, 2010). I have grouped them under the headings of establishing the therapeutic alliance; the nonverbal processes of listening and containing; the implementation of therapeutic limits; and the mastery of verbal communications, such as expressions of attunement, invitations to elaborate, clarifications of issues, exposures of self-defeating patterns, and interpretations of meaning.

Establishing the Therapeutic Alliance

Clinicians new to psychoanalytic therapies often start trying to "do therapy" without sufficiently explaining the process to patients. Especially now, with the ascendency of treatments characterized by practitioner-directed strategies rather than mutual exploration and a stance of not knowing, and when the surrounding culture offers few accurate images of psychoanalytic work, beginners need to know how to explain psychodynamic therapy to patients. These days, they will often be asked by patients directly at the beginning of treatment, "How does this work?"

They need to be armed with potential responses to such queries. Supervisors can rehearse with them ways of describing the analytic process. Such explications might involve the following elements:

1. We need to understand the problem in some depth before moving to solutions.

2. I am assuming that the interpersonal patterns that brought you here will eventually become a part of your relationship with me.

3. By addressing your problematic patterns safely here, you will acquire new ways of understanding and dealing with them.

4. You may need to mourn some painful past experiences before you can reduce their hold on you.

Supervisees should be prepared for possible explanatory work later in the treatment as well. Otherwise, feeling muzzled by what they understand to be "standard technique," they may become stiff and anxious when patients confront them about what is going on. For example, when clinicians begin to ask clients about possible transference reactions, they may need to explain again that they are asking because they are trying to probe here-and-now experiences for what they reveal about patterns in the patient's life. Or when a patient asks a question that is better explored than answered, they should be prepared to respond that although they very much want to hear the patient's questions, they may choose not to answer them, because in this kind of treatment it is more important to learn why a particular question has arisen and what it reveals about the client's underlying concerns. When responding to the content of a question might move the work forward, the supervisor can suggest saying, "I will be glad to answer your question, but first, let's explore why it is coming up now and what are the thoughts and feelings behind it." Supervisees appreciate having this response ready in their repertoire.

Supervisors also need to help novice psychodynamic therapists to deal with issues involving diagnosis. Because third parties who support treatments require diagnostic labels, because it is a patient's legal right to know the diagnoses of record, and because patients may feel infantilized or alarmed when they feel a therapist hedges about a diagnostic question, clinicians need to learn how to describe, in respectful and commonsense ways, conditions that in popular parlance are often stigmatized, for example, bipolar disorder, borderline personality disorder, or psychosis. Individuals who come to treatment describing themselves by less frightening labels—for instance, those who explain that they have a social phobia or an eating disorder—often ask either early or later in treatment, "Do I have a personality disorder? Which one?"

Mentors can help their students with how to talk about the limits of categorical psychiatric diagnoses and how to involve patients in an exploration of the concerns behind their questions. My own supervisees have been surprised to learn that, in an effort to demonstrate that I am not keeping any potentially dangerous secrets from them, I have sometimes given patients the DSM, and asked which personality disorder seems closest to how they see themselves. In my experience, they almost always choose the most apt category, opening the way to my asking about specific instances when they behaved in certain ways or demonstrated certain traits. They tend to feel respected by this gesture, and I think it helps to strengthen the alliance.

Finally, the supervisor may need to help supervisees obtain truly informed consent for treatment, including knowledge of the limits of confidentiality and other potentially problematic areas, without setting a tone that makes the arrangements sound too fussy. They will need to be sure the patient understands policies involving fees, cancellations, and other areas that newer clinicians often minimize because of their discomfort with setting limits, a topic I talk about shortly. All these activities at the beginning of treatment contribute to the safety and comfort of the working alliance. Given the critical contribution of this element to the success of treatment (Flückiger, Del Re, Wampold, Symonds, & Horvath, 2012; Krupnick et al., 2006; Levendosky & Hopwood, 2016; Safran & Muran, 2003), supervisors should be sure that the clinician knows to ask, toward the end of an initial interview, about whether the patient feels comfortable with the prospect of working together. This question also sets the stage for the "you-and-me" talk that will follow, as the therapist investigates the transference–countertransference situation. The establishment of a good supervisory alliance will have helped the clinician in this direction.

Listening and Containing

The hardest psychodynamic skill is simply *listening* in a way that encourages clients to keep talking so that the therapist can get a sense of the associative networks behind the patient's experience. Encouraging free association or speaking as freely as possible allows psychoanalytic therapists to hear the themes and rhythms of the patient's inner life and to extract less conscious meanings from the manifest content of the person's communications. This attitude does not come naturally to human beings when we are in contact with someone who is suffering or who relates a horrific experience. We normally respond with a reference to comparable events we have endured, or we give advice or reassurance, or we change the subject because it is too painful to stay on topic. With our patients, we have to learn the art of asking for more details and more elaboration when they share their miseries with us. Simply asking them. "Can you say more about that?" is a lot more useful than our typical social responses.

Psychological evaluation instruments can be very valuable to therapists and patients. There are numerous assessment procedures available to clinicians that are useful for formulating treatment types and goals; sometimes I refer patients for psychological testing by colleagues who are better trained than I am in that area. Because administering psychological tests is beyond my own scope of practice, I do not highlight this kind of supervision in this book. But I do want to observe that new therapists, especially those trained in psychology, may rush defensively to such instruments, avoiding the intense affects that can fill the consulting room when a patient begins to describe psychological pain. Posing open-ended queries tends to be more immediately evocative than having clients endorse DSM criteria for particular diagnoses or fill out assessment forms. Therapists who are too eager to give patients objective tests risk cutting off important information. Supervisors often have to help them be more still and receptive. Or, as the great researcher Hans Strupp was reportedly fond of saying, "Don't just do something, sit there!" (T. Schact, listserv communication, May 2, 2020).

Helping patients talk about their experience involves many skills, including the capacity to tolerate silence. Being quiet long enough for the patient to reflect and then fill the silent space is difficult, especially for those of us in cultures that reward extroversion (see Cain, 2012). There are many different kinds of silences, though; some feel hostile, others express hopelessness, some stem from fear or from shame, some express an internal conflict, and some result from a patient's lack of words for an emotional experience. Depending on the most probable meaning of a patient's silence, it is not always right for a therapist to be quiet in response. But when it is, it is important that the clinician be comfortable with a stillness that would be out of place in nonclinical situations.

In ordinary social discourse, we are also not highly self-conscious about our facial expressions. With friends, relatives, colleagues, and acquaintances, the degree to which we have to monitor our face, body language, and general appearance is significantly lower than with clients. In therapy, the discipline of containment (Bion, 1962) is directly related to how freely a patient can talk. Some fascinating work has been done in Germany by Rainer Krause and his colleagues (e.g., Anstadt, Merten, Ullrich, & Krause, 1997) on therapists' facial affect and patient responses. Studies with real patients seeing experienced therapists (in contrast to much research done in the United States, which tends to depend on student therapists and patients with one DSM disorder without comorbidities) have shown that even "treatment-resistant" clients make significant therapeutic progress when they see facial expressions in their therapists that differ markedly from those they expect or typically evoke in others. For example, the patient expects anger, and the therapist's face shows curiosity; or the patient expects contempt, and the therapist looks angry that someone shamed the patient; or the patient expects disgust, and the therapist's face shows sadness.

I think most clinicians know the importance of facial expression intuitively and consequently put considerable conscious and unconscious effort into their nonverbal transmissions. They try to maintain a warm, interested demeanor, often despite feeling a swirl of other less attractive reactions to the patient's communications. Face monitoring is not a skill that supervisors tend to teach explicitly, but they do model it, permitting newer therapists to learn it by identification. In my book on diagnosis (McWilliams, 2011), I mentioned the subspecialty skill of the "nose yawn." The number of colleagues who have told me that this concept resonated with them is impressive. It appears that clinicians recognize this kind of struggle over what we convey nonverbally in the clinical role. In addition to exemplifying professional equanimity, supervisors may have to help their mentees adapt to, and vent about, how tiring it can be to maintain a benign countenance.

Setting Limits

The second hardest skill involves *limit setting*. All clinical practice depends on some clarity between therapist and client about the conditions under which the clinician can work comfortably and the patient can pursue change. But setting limits that are vital for therapeutic progress can be difficult, especially when one is working with someone who feels emotionally desperate, needy, and deeply resentful of reasonable constraints. Many graduate and postgraduate programs give this critical area short shrift, and even when they do address it, the complexities of limit setting are not really alive to students until they arise in the clinical situation.

Newer therapists need help with dilemmas as simple as how to get a distressed and clingy patient out the door kindly at the end of the session. They need specifics about how they might respond to clients who offer them expensive gifts, or insist on a hug, or invite them to weddings, funerals, or graduations. They need to find graceful, nonpunitive ways to deal with requests for personal information, pressures from parents for explicit details of their child's sessions, and demands from attorneys for information to be used in litigation. With some patients, clinical work feels like an endless process of saying no as gently and firmly as possible. Many therapists are natural people pleasers, and beginners in this field are not used to imposing limits on others.

In this area of maintaining the therapeutic frame, supervisees are helped by examples of contracts covering policies about payment, cancellations, no-shows, confidentiality and its limits, and so on. They need suggestions about how to remind clients tactfully about mutually agreed-upon goals of treatment and how to look at what may be in the way of their making progress with them. They need to learn how to cope with patients who fail to pay their bills or who receive insurance reimbursement and pocket the money instead of paying the clinician. With more disturbed patients, they may need to remind them of the agreements they have made with respect to self-destructive behaviors, including attempts at suicide (see, e.g., Caligor, Kernberg, Clarkin, & Yeomans, 2018).

Supervisees who intend to write about clinical experiences need mentoring about the process of getting permission from patients whose treatment they discuss and/or about adequately disguising clinical material. They may need to be alerted to the probable therapeutic consequences of patients' permission (or lack of permission) for the clinician to write about them, and they may need help with addressing the emotional aftermath, once the person's inevitably mixed feelings about being written about emerge in treatment. Again, this attention to less conscious negative reactions to the therapist is a distinguishing characteristic and vital wellspring of psychoanalytic work.

Verbal Communications

The third area in which specific skills need to be taught involves verbal interventions, specifically, the timing, tone, and content of comments intended to communicate empathy, address defenses, make connections, or infer meaning from a patient's material. Students need to learn that one can be brilliantly astute and not at all therapeutic. Clinical progress has very little to do with a therapist's being "right," a reality that can be hard for supervisees to take in when most of their previous educational successes have involved demonstrating to authorities that they have the correct answer. Beginning clinicians need to know that what satisfied clients remember and value about their treatments is not their therapist's dazzling interpretations. Instead, they recall the therapist's overall attitude of warmth, hope, interest, and respect (e.g., Leamy, Bird, Le Boutillier, & Williams, 2011).

Still, what one says to patients does matter. Verbal communications can make people feel deeply understood, moved, curious to learn more, challenged to be their best selves, and grateful for insight. They can also do harm: They can make a client feel shamed, blamed, or patronized; they can shut down self-exploration and self-exposure; they can inadvertently teach the lesson that one doesn't have to work on oneself, that one can simply depend on the brilliant therapist. Supervisors need to help clinicians have reasonable criteria for judging whether what they have said has maximized their therapeutic effectiveness or, contrastingly, created pain and resistance to hearing more (Strupp, Hadley, & Gomez-Schwartz, 1977). From their mentors, therapists need both modeling and thoughtful suggestions about what they can say when confronting various clinical challenges.

NURTURING ETHICAL SENSIBILITIES

In addition to helping mentees develop the previous skills, supervisors are responsible for helping them translate ethical standards from theory into practice. Medical professionals regard taking the Hippocratic oath as a sacred ritual. Clinical, counseling, and social work programs typically focus on educating their students about ethical issues, both general principles and specific implementations appropriate to their discipline. The ethics code of the American Psychological Association (2017), for example, foregrounds the principles of beneficence, fidelity/responsibility, integrity, justice, and respect for people's rights and dignity. The Association's code of conduct specifies the application of these principles to professional behavior; for example, do not have sex with patients, avoid dual roles, do not make exceptions for confidentiality except as required by law, do not practice beyond your sphere of competence.

Beginning therapists need to have (and most do have) both an intellectual mastery of this territory and also a more personally integrated "feel" for the clinical implications of the code of ethics in their discipline. The real-life applications of these principles will become much more vivid to them when patients confront them with ethical dilemmas in the here and now. Even though a reputable training program will have approached ethics training via vignettes that promote discussion of clinical choice points, the lived experience of such choice points can feel strikingly different from, and more challenging than, the hypothetical situations discussed in class. The emotional pressure in the clinical moment and the intensity of transference and countertransference cannot easily be created prospectively by role playing in class. Supervision is the ideal setting in which to learn to steer one's ethical ship while riding out the storms of clinical engagement.

Some supervisees are so concerned with being pragmatically and morally above criticism, so fixed on seeing themselves as conforming to high professional standards, that they approach both practical and ethical issues concretely, with an obsessive determination to find the "rule" that applies to every clinical situation. They need a supervisor's help in becoming more comfortable with the fact that no clinical rule book can cover every potential real-world challenge. All of us in the mental health field take a long time in evolving toward feeling and behaving more like responsible adults than compliant (or rebellious) children.

We need to use judgment, wisdom, and reflection with respect to the principles that underlie particular ethical stipulations. We need to consider whether two or more principles may be in conflict and to imagine the probable outcomes of different solutions to clinical problems. As my colleague Russ Healy has noted, in this field we tend to start out being principlists ("What basic rule should I follow?") and end up being consequentialists ("What will likely be the outcome of my doing this?"). In interviews with elderly psychoanalytic therapists widely admired for their clinical wisdom, Cynthia Baum-Baicker found that they spontaneously mentioned certain common themes: openness to experience, capacity to tolerate uncertainty and paradox, sensitivity to complexity, respect for conventional rules coexisting with a willingness to challenge them, and a sense of balance between immersion in experience and critical reflection (Baum-Baicker & Sisti, 2012). This combination is what we want to nurture in supervisees.

Clinical wisdom is rarely simple. When faced with treatment quandaries, supervisees need mentorship to get them into the habit of asking their patients for time to think about any question that makes them uncomfortable. This simple buying of time can help liberate them from the stress of immediate dilemmas. Knowing they can say, "Let me think about that; I'll get back to you next time with my thoughts" provides space for reflection when the emotional pressure is on. It allows therapists to expose the clinical situation to someone who will not feel the same countertransference intensity. Young practitioners should be made aware that this need to take a pause and ask for help never goes away over the course of one's career. Whenever one feels conflicted about what is the "right" thing to do (or, more typically, the "better" thing to do, since most clinical decisions have pros and cons), one should ideally consult someone else: a more experienced therapist, a specialist in a particular area, a supervision group, a legal advisor.

Most professional organizations have ethical boards, committees, or specialists whose job it is to confer with therapists facing clinical dilemmas. Insurance companies, concerned with the possible financial consequences of therapists' mistakes, typically employ risk management advisors who can be helpful. If there is ever a complaint made against a clinician, the fact that the therapist has consulted with other professionals is a mitigating factor in the decisions of the professional boards that hear such cases. Newer therapists often harbor the fantasy that if they are truly competent, they should be making difficult decisions by themselves with skill and confidence. Supervisors need to break it to them kindly that this fantasy will never be realized.

Because it is a core supervisory responsibility to ensure that the clinicians we train will do no harm (Alonso, 1985), and also because I find ethical issues more challenging in supervision than in psychotherapy, I devote Chapter 6 to questions about our responsibilities as supervisors to the larger community and its values. There I give several lengthy examples of efforts to help supervisees with questions of ethics. But for purposes of this overview, let me note that as in other areas of supervision, exemplifying a stance is more pedagogically powerful than teaching about it. Acting with integrity in "small" matters (writing reference letters on time, returning phone calls within a day, not canceling sessions casually, giving ample notice of upcoming breaks) and in big ones (being honest with the supervisee, observing norms of confidentiality) is more important than teaching about it.

SOCIALIZING SUPERVISEES INTO A PSYCHOANALYTIC ETHOS

All the supervisory procedures listed in this chapter contribute to what Brenner and Khan (2013) have described as the training of supervisees

in "psychoanalytic virtue." Although their target audience for this formulation is physicians overseeing medical residents in psychiatry, their
observations apply to training in any domain of psychoanalytic practice.
Their list of distinctively psychodynamic virtues includes empathy; neutrality and affirmation (meaning, by neutrality, Anna Freud's concept
of equidistance from the id, ego, and superego, rather than later equa-
tions of the term with nonresponsiveness); a conviction that meaning lies
ahead; the embrace of complexity, uncertainty, and humility; openness
to transference; and avoiding the gratifications to the therapist's narcissism that can come with being more authoritative or attuning preferen-
tially to the patient's positive feelings.

In mentoring aspiring psychodynamic therapists and psychoanalysts, supervisors are essentially welcoming them into a community with
its own guiding set of values. Roy Shafer gave his version of this sensibility in his 1983 book, *The Analytic Attitude*. I have described other
elements of the psychoanalytic ethos in a book on therapy (McWilliams,
2004) and in an article on Jeremy Safran's work (McWilliams, 2019).
Sandra Buechler (2004) has similarly described orienting psychoanalytic
values, depicting them in terms of emotions that guide psychoanalytic
treatment. These frames of reference may be quite different from the
utilitarian, pragmatic approaches that supervisees may have previously
absorbed, and although they function mostly silently, they are a critical
part of psychoanalytic supervision.

STIMULATING ONGOING CURIOSITY
AND PREVENTING BURNOUT

One of the benefits I cherish most about a psychoanalytic perspective
is that it makes clinical work continually interesting. An appreciation
of the overdetermination of symptoms, the extent of unconscious conflict, the inevitability of internalizing multifaceted others, the layering
of defensive processes, the complexity of emotion, and the power of
subtle nonverbal processes guarantees that there is always something in
a clinical encounter that can evoke one's curiosity or awake one's compassion. Even when a supervisee is working with a boring or devaluing
client, mentor and mentee can become intrigued together about how
the person became so psychologically empty. Supervisors who grasp the
immensity of unconscious processes and the complexity of individual
solutions to life's problems tend to exemplify un-self-consciously the

vitality inherent in a psychodynamic perspective and lay the ground-work for their supervisees' pleasure in lifelong learning (see, e.g., Aggarwal & Bhatia, 2020).

If I had been trained in a series of manualized interventions for specific symptom syndromes, I think I would have burned out early in my career. After almost half a century in psychoanalytic practice, I am still enlivened by its exploratory nature and its capacity to surprise. As I learn from patients about the infinite ways in which they perceive and engage with their lives, my own world expands and my capacity for mentalization increases. For people of my general temperament, analytic therapy and supervision are inherently creative and satisfying. I have colleagues in their eighties and nineties who continue to see clients not because they need the money but because they love the work.

Because all therapists care about helping people, and because this work is not easy to do, clinicians of all theoretical orientations may over-extend themselves, chafe at the limitations of their settings, feel defeated by their patients' life problems, and suffer compassion fatigue and secondary traumatization. Burnout is thus an occupational hazard for all of us, and new learning is a fine antidote to getting stale and demoralized in any clinical arena (see, e.g., Boyd-Franklin, Cleek, Wofsky, & Mundy, 2015). It is my prejudice, however, that because of the fascination inherent in an in-depth understanding of clinical challenges, burnout is less of a problem for psychodynamically oriented clinicians than for others (this would be an interesting proposition to test empirically). Analytic supervisors naturally model ongoing learning and set the stage for life-long nourishment of the mind and heart.

WHAT PSYCHOANALYTIC SUPERVISION IS NOT

I began this chapter by making some generalizations about good supervision. I cannot resist ending it with a few words about bad supervision, that is, about what does not belong in any approach to training in the psychodynamic therapies: Supervision should not involve indoctrination, bullying, or the exploitation of an opportunity to absorb the idealization of the vulnerable. These cautions would not be necessary if I had not heard many stories of such crimes being committed in the name of psychoanalysis (see also Ellis, 2017; Ellis et al., 2014). Here is a relevant anecdote offered spontaneously by my colleague Mary Lamia when she learned that I was working on a book on psychoanalytic supervision:

I am reminded of a supervisor during my psychoanalytic training who *insisted* [original emphasis] that I interpret my patient's erotic transference that was not in the least bit overt. For many reasons, I had felt strongly that the patient was not ready to hear such an interpretation and would respond negatively to it. My supervisor eventually told me that if I didn't interpret the erotic transference, I would end up with a poor evaluation from him. Hence, I delivered the interpretation in the most gentle way possible. The patient said, "I'm not going to go there," and he left treatment. To this day, over 30 years later, I still wish I could apologize to that patient or go back in time and sacrifice my analytic training for the sake of his treatment. It haunts me.

I would guess that most of us have a horror story of this sort. It is not uncommon for us to rue the consequences, long after the fact, of submitting to a dominating supervisor. In this case, even if the supervisor was right about the patient's erotic fantasies about the therapist, he could not have reasonably expected her to be able to convey such an interpretation effectively without feeling some sense of comfort with conveying that message. And, with a dose of humility, he might have considered the additional possibility that she was right and he was wrong.

In my experience, analytic supervisors are generally respectful of the fact that it is the supervisee, not the supervisor, who is "in the room" with the client (cf. Yerushalmi, 2018). It is the supervisee who is getting the most accurate nonverbal data about what is possible and not possible to say at any given point. But some of us evidently cannot get past a tendency to throw our weight around or show off our assumed superior understanding. We need to remember that even when we are sure we know better than the supervisee, unless there is a pressing ethical issue involved, we cannot effectively induce a supervisee to move past what is visible to him or her in the clinical situation, and we should not push our less experienced colleagues beyond their comfort zones—especially not through power-play threats to give them bad evaluations, as this supervisor did with Dr. Lamia.

CONCLUDING COMMENTS

In this chapter, I have summarized what I have come to see as the functions of a good analytic supervisor, including offering support, promoting honesty, providing information, teaching skills, nurturing ethical sensibilities, and modeling ongoing learning that will prevent burnout.

I have put particular emphasis on the lifelong need of clinicians for self-reflection and consultation. This overview only ripples the surface of the deep reservoir that constitutes thoughtful and useful psychoanalytic supervision. In subsequent parts of this book, I take up more specific issues. The next chapter explores the history of psychoanalytic supervision, with a special focus on recurring themes and issues that have arisen over more than a century of inducting less experienced colleagues into our peculiar art.

Chapter Two

■ ■ ■ ■

Historical Background
of Psychoanalytic Supervision

How to teach psychodynamic psychotherapy to students and interested professionals, how to support and increase clinical competence as therapists mature, how to prevent or repair conduct that is unhelpful (or outright hurtful) to patients, and how to ensure that clinicians keep learning and growing throughout their careers have been recurrent issues in mental health education for well over a century. Like most topics in the psychotherapy literature, the professional conversation about these matters began with Sigmund Freud. Let me start there.

FREUD'S CONTRIBUTIONS

Freud said very little explicitly about psychoanalytic supervision. But he approached the question implicitly from three directions: the experiential, the intellectual, and the ethical. (One could thus frame his overall contribution, although he did not, as attending to the respective realms of the id, ego, and superego.) First, he argued that all professionals who want to practice psychoanalysis should go through analysis themselves. Second, he described the clinical techniques that had worked for him, along with his rationale for having adopted them. Third, he articulated ethical concerns that he felt should guide the profession. These elements remain central to supervision. Ideally, supervisors want to turn out therapists who (1) have a deep, organic feeling for the work and confidence in its value, (2) have cognitive mastery of the theoretical, clinical, and empirical literatures that guide it, and (3) practice with integrity.

Like almost all analysts who came after him, Freud (e.g., 1926) viewed the first tenet as self-evident, perhaps comparable to a music teacher's conviction that the best way to learn melody, harmony, and rhythm is to immerse oneself in music. In their own treatments, he noted, therapists would have intimate experience with intense transferences and anxiety-based resistances to change, and they would learn firsthand about the power of unconscious fantasies, wishes, and fears. They would also become aware of their own blind spots and be less likely to miss comparable areas in patients. Psychoanalysis is essentially an educative process that potentiates personal maturation (McWilliams, 2003), and the role of analyst requires an unusual degree of emotional sensitivity and self-awareness.

Of all the statements Freud made about how to become a good or better practitioner, his belief that those of us who intend to be therapists need our own treatment is probably the most universally endorsed principle among psychodynamically oriented clinicians. This conviction is shared across the diverse theoretical preferences and background disciplines that make up the psychoanalytic community. As far as I know, personal therapy is required by all psychoanalytic institutes. In informal surveys, graduates of analytic training programs often rank their personal analyses as the most valuable part of their clinical education, their supervision as the second most vital influence, and their course work a somewhat distant third. The norm of therapy for the therapist was adopted by the humanistic tradition in psychotherapy and has been subjected to empirical investigations that have supported its value (see Geller, Norcross, & Orlinsky, 2005).

Freud (1911a, 1912a, 1912b, 1913, 1914, 1915) explicated the second area mostly in his papers on technique. He did so relatively early in his career as a therapist, about 2 decades after his original work with patients suffering from the dissociative symptoms that were at the time called hysteria, but before he had developed and refined his more mature ideas. When he wrote the technique essays, a point at which increasing numbers of his colleagues were becoming interested in his method, he seems to have been responding to entreaties to give specifics about how he worked. Most of his recommendations were offered with a notable lack of dogmatism. For example, he wrote in his 1912b paper: "This technique is the only one suited to my individuality; I do not venture to deny that a physician quite differently constituted might find himself driven to adopt a different attitude to his patients and to the task before him" (p. 111). And in his 1913 paper, he carefully noted:

> I think I am well-advised . . . to call these rules "recommenda-
> tions" and not to claim any unconditional acceptance for them.
> The extraordinary diversity of the psychical constellations con-
> cerned, the plasticity of all mental processes and the wealth of
> determining factors oppose any mechanization of the technique;
> and they bring it about that a course of action that is as a rule
> justified may at times prove ineffective, whilst one that is usually
> mistaken may once in a while lead to the desired end. (p. 123)

Despite this open-minded stance, many of Freud's statements about how he worked were received by his admirers as the last word on technique. When supervising others, some of his more doctrinaire followers saw it as their proper role to confront students about every instance when they were not practicing exactly as the Master had recommended. This supervisory style—the psychoanalytic equivalent of putting more emphasis on following the manual than understanding the therapeutic process—seems rare now among analysts, at least in the United States, but it was not uncommon in the mid-20th century, and in many communities, it gave analytic training a bad name. It is not a version of psychoanalytic supervision that informs this book, which comports more closely with Freud's ideas about adapting to individuality, both one's own and that of the patient.

In the area of ethics, Freud was unequivocal in urging his colleagues not to exploit their patients, sexually and otherwise. In the early years of psychoanalysis, when patriarchal authority and entitlement were taken for granted, and when analysts were only beginning to learn how their role attracted intense reenactments of childhood traumas and fantasies, this position of "No, not ever!" was more radical than it may seem in hindsight (Gabbard, 1995). Freud committed many clinical errors, including some we would now consider ethical violations (such as his analyzing his daughter Anna or meddling in the love life of his patient and friend Sándor Ferenczi), but he was ethically ahead of his time on the issue of sex between patient and therapist. Many of his peers were not so clearheaded. Sexual violations by early analysts were not uncommon and have been well documented (e.g., Berman & Mosher, 2019). The wheedling but adamant tone of Freud's messages on this topic suggests that he was trying to persuade colleagues not to do what they were already doing. Gabbard (1995) notes his distress about the sexually exploitive acts that Carl Jung and Ernest Jones, among others, were then rationalizing.

In a related ethical area, Freud urged therapists to resist temptations to act as "prophet, saviour and redeemer to the patient" (1923, p. 50). In other words, he took a dim view of using clients to bolster one's self-image as sexually desirable or as intellectually or morally superior. At a time when many of his colleagues had what we now see as dreadful boundaries, when some had a tendency to promise their patients salvation through their brilliant grasp of the "new science" of psychoanalysis, Freud was prescient in seeing the danger inherent in promising more from analytic therapy than it can realistically deliver. The ethical directive not to practice beyond one's area of competence is a contemporary echo of this position.

Over Freud's long career, it is noteworthy how little he said about training. This omission may be a good thing, as it opened psychoanalysis up to diverse perspectives on the education of therapists, conversations that may not have happened if Freud had taken an authoritarian position on supervision. For many decades, professionals in supervisory roles were working out, by trial and error, approaches that seemed to be effective for them. As psychodynamic therapy has evolved, through both clinical experience and empirical research, we have come to conceptualize supervision in increasingly complex and sophisticated ways.

We have also become less self-deluded and naïve. Many American psychoanalytic institutes in the first decades of the 20th century required the analysts of their candidates to comment on the psychological maturity of the aspiring graduate (see Lifschutz, 1976, for an early commentary, and Wallerstein, 2010, for a historical review of this practice, which continued in some cases into the 1980s). Although this convention of "reporting analysts" makes sense superficially, it is ludicrous psychologically. How could such "analyses" have been remotely therapeutic? If one is aware that one's analyst has to report to institute authorities, how can one not keep secrets, consciously or unconsciously? Institutes do need to have procedures for evaluating candidates and weeding out those who are personally or ethically unsuited to the work, but psychoanalysis itself depends on truly free association (cf. Kairys, 1964). I mention this bizarre chapter in analytic history of the "reporting analyst," which has not entirely ended in some locales, because a related problem about information sharing, one without an easy solution, arises in many supervisory situations. I address this issue later in this chapter and elsewhere.

POST-FREUDIAN CONTRIBUTIONS

For many years after Freud's death, much psychoanalytic supervision was fairly authoritarian, concerning itself with teaching therapists the "rules" of psychoanalytic procedure. The original standards for psychoanalytic training, delineated by Max Eitingon in 1923 (the "Eitingon model" or "Berlin model"), emphasized the transmission of knowledge more than the goal of supporting the supervisee's autonomy, creativity, and personal development. The more relational elements of learning how to be a competent therapist were assumed to come from one's personal analysis. There were many exceptions to this generalization, as individual supervisors developed their own styles, but there was not much scholarly theorizing about more nuanced ways of construing the supervisory process. My impression, based on conversations with older analysts, is that until toward the end of the last century, some supervisors who worked more relationally found themselves characterized as "deviating" from a professional norm.

The first systematic study of clinical supervision was a landmark work by Rudolf Ekstein and Robert Wallerstein (1958/1971). In their investigation, reported in a book that is still worth reading despite its somewhat archaic language and its focus on psychiatrists in medical settings, parallels emerged between the patient–clinician relationship and the clinician–supervisor relationship. Specifically, the supervisors they studied found themselves feeling and behaving in ways that uncannily mirrored the feelings, attitudes, and behaviors of their supervisee toward the patient who was being discussed. This finding attracted attention to what Ekstein and Wallerstein felicitously called the "parallel process," a phenomenon that Harold Searles (1955) had previously observed and termed a "reflection process." Parenthetically, while Ekstein and Wallerstein were squarely in the psychoanalytic mainstream, the more maverick Searles, whose writing was remarkably self-exposing for his buttoned-up era, had a strong influence on the generation of analysts who came of age in the less conformist 1960s (see, e.g., Ogden, 2005).

In the parallel process, the countertransference of a therapist toward a patient unconsciously evokes a similar attitude in the supervisor toward the therapist. Contemporary analysts would ascribe this phenomenon to the mental operations that Melanie Klein (1946) called projective identification and/or attribute it to right-brain-to-right-brain communication processes (Schore, 2019). Since the 1950s, the parallel process has been extensively documented, both anecdotally and empirically (Baudry, 1993; Caligor, 1981; Doehrman, 1976; Gediman & Wolkenfeld, 1980;

Miller & Twomey, 1999; Nagell, Steinmetzer, Fissabre, & Spilski, 2014; Perlman, 1996; Sarnat, 2019; Searles, 1955, 1962; Tracey, Bludworth, & Glidden-Tracey, 2012; Watkins, 2017).

In 1966, Fleming and Benedek wrote an influential book about supervision, grounded in the study of audiotaped sessions. Although the supervision of their era was generally more patriarchal in tone, they introduced the critical concept of the "learning alliance." They argued that what goes on in supervision is much more interpersonally complex than the transmission of skills from a more competent to a less competent person. This observation presaged an eventual psychoanalytic emphasis on the supervisory process itself and on the nature of the supervisory relationship, not just on the content of the supervisor's teaching (see Frawley-O'Dea & Sarnat, 2001; Szecsödy, 1989, 2008). Along with the now widely appreciated parallel process that Ekstein and Wallerstein had observed traveling unconsciously from patient to therapist to supervisor, the analytic community gradually recognized that similar processes can work in the other direction. A harshly critical supervisor, for example, can unwittingly influence a supervisee to be harshly critical toward a client (see, e.g., Eagle & Long, 2014).

By the end of the 20th century, more authoritarian models of supervision had been replaced in most psychoanalytic communities by a relational model, in which the development of a positive supervisory alliance was given more emphasis than the teaching of particular clinical techniques (Berman, 2000; Frawley-O'Dea & Sarnat, 2001; Watkins, 2015a). By the last third of the 20th century, variations in supervisory style were so evident that Edgar Levenson (1982) described six models of psychoanalytic supervision, all embodying different interpersonal dynamics, which he whimsically dubbed "holding or confirming," "Teutonic or by-the-numbers," "algorithmic," "metatherapeutic," "zen," and "preceptorship."

C. E. Watkins, Jr. (2011, 2015a, 2015c, 2016, 2017) has reviewed this relational evolution, framing it as a movement "from pedagogical to andragogical" supervision, the latter being defined by the following features:

> (1) the supervisor is assigned responsibility as a learning facilitator or educational change agent; (2) the supervisee is viewed as an adult learner par excellence, actively involved in the entirety of the learning experience and making it optimally beneficial; (3) power and influence are shared by the co-participants, and (4) mutual respect is preponderant in their relationship. (2015a, p. 234)

These elements comprise a pithy summary of the current clinical consensus about the proper nature of psychoanalytic supervision, amounting to a shift in emphasis from authoritatively didactic to mutually experiential. As Watkins (2011) has noted, although this evolution began in psychoanalysis, has ebbed and flowed, has been gradual, and remains incomplete, at this point the professional emphasis on the supervisory relationship has become axiomatic and transtheoretical; that is, the assumption of the importance of the relationship in supervision is shared by humanistic, cognitive, and systems-oriented therapists.

RECURRENT THEMES AND TENSIONS

Among the controversies that have reappeared with some regularity in the analytic literature on supervision are the questions of whether the supervisor should "teach or treat" and whether one should emphasize imparting skills or fostering general professional maturation (see Watkins, 2011). There has also been some conflict about whether one's own analyst should also be one's supervisor, either during one's analysis or after it. Let me start with that issue, which has been more or less resolved over time but has echoes in current practice.

The Question of the Supervisor's Proper Role

In the early days of psychoanalysis, a contrast emerged between the "Berlin model" explicated by Max Eitingon and the "Hungarian" or "Budapest" model of training, championed by Sándor Ferenczi (Kovacs, 1936; Perlman, 1996; Rachman, 2016). Briefly, the convention in the Berlin professional community was to ask would-be analysts to seek supervision from sources other than their own analyst. Proponents of this view were sensitive to the danger that a novice clinician might overidentify with one professional or approach at the expense of developing a personal integration of different styles. They also noted that when analysts became supervisors to their former patients, they risked depriving them of an uncontaminated therapeutic relationship to which they could return if they found themselves needing psychological help in the future.

The Hungarian group had a more relaxed attitude about combining roles. Their essential argument was, "Who better than the personal analyst to know a practitioner's vulnerabilities and strengths?" They felt that the deep knowledge an analyst had of an analysand's personality could only be an advantage in zeroing in tactfully on what the new clinician needed to work on. It was also assumed that by the time they were treating patients, aspiring analysts would have attained a level of maturity and comfort with being known intimately, "warts and all," that would enable them to tolerate the analyst's evaluative comments without yielding to a temptation to withhold negative information. During their therapeutic experience, it was assumed, they would also have become free to challenge the analyst if they disagreed with a supervisory suggestion. The legacy of the Budapest group includes our increasing sensitivity to the inevitable interpenetration of supervision with therapeutic growth, as well as our growing appreciation of the complicated, intersubjective emotional field within which supervisor and supervisee do their work (see Berman, 2000; Soreanu, 2019; Wilner, 2015).

This early disagreement about the boundary conditions of supervision was at least partly an artifact of a time when analysts were scarce: One's own therapist might be the most—or even the only—fully trained psychoanalyst in town. Being both treated and taught by the same trainee of Freud or one of his protégés was virtually inescapable. But as more people pursued a psychoanalytic education, and as some complications of practitioners' inhabiting dual roles became apparent, members of the analytic community have reached some consensus on the value of differentiating analyst from supervisor, in line with the Berlin rather than the Budapest model. Specifically, Eitingon's (1926) recommendation that the personal analysis be separate from the more apprenticeship-like experience of supervision has become the norm (see Watkins, 2013a). There remain some individual differences among supervisors on this question, however.

The issue of professionals playing dual roles plagues supervision contemporarily and has been noted in the supervision literature at least since the pioneering work of Fleming and Benedek (1966). It has not arisen so much in the area of whether a therapist's own therapist should give supervisory comments, but with respect to a different problem: Teachers of psychotherapy seek from their supervisees a completely honest relationship despite the fact that if the supervisees are still in training, supervisors are expected to evaluate them candidly to those who will decide on their progress through a graduate or postgraduate program. In fact, "gatekeeping" is one of the sacred obligations of practitioners in any human services profession.

Evaluative obligations apply only rarely when clinicians are already beyond the gate (i.e., when they have already been credentialed as independent practitioners). Similarly, they may not apply when therapists work for an agency that has the legal responsibility to oversee their work, if such clinicians have independently hired an outside consultant for their personal development who has no institutional accountability. But the obligation to protect the public from incompetent or unethical practitioners complicates the supervisory process in graduate training.

One way to reduce the psychological complexities is for an academic faculty to appoint supervisors in the community who are not professors in the training program. These clinicians do have to evaluate students, but only on their response to supervision. Professors of trainees in clinical and counseling programs have much wider oversight responsibility for student progress, and that reality interferes with students' comfort in reporting with complete candor on their clinical work. For this reason, my graduate students at Rutgers University have tended to prefer outside supervisors to those on the academic faculty. To an external supervisor, they can complain about their training program and in other ways be more candid than they could be with a professor who has some responsibility for endorsing their readiness to graduate. Yet not every program can easily find or afford enough experienced external mentors and, in such instances, supervision falls to the teaching faculty. I say more about this situation and its complexities in later chapters.

To Teach or to Treat?

The "teach or treat" problem is an interesting one, and probably a somewhat artificial dichotomy. As early as 1955, there was a spirited discussion about the topic on an American Psychoanalytic Association panel (Sloane, 1957), with views all over the map. Cabaniss and colleagues (2001) have a nice review of the teach-versus-treat question, concluding that although most supervising analysts stay out of the role of treater, there continues to be wide individual variation in how people supervise, especially in how free the supervisor feels to go into the emotional life of the supervisee. They rightly note the paucity of empirical data on this topic (this is beginning to change, but is still very much the case).

I know of numerous instances in which an analytic supervisor seems to have treated a supervisee too much like a patient and too little like a mentee (e.g., responding to requests for supervisory help with queries about the supervisee's feelings, or relating all clinical problems to the student's family background, or inquiring intrusively into disclosures of any history of trauma, or postulating inferred dynamics in the supervisee without asking permission to speculate in this way). This approach does not usually go well, especially early in one's training. Beginning therapists generally feel too vulnerable to expose their soft subjective underbellies (cf. Zicht, 2019). Realistically, no matter how much the current practice of supervision has focused on examining subjective experience, novice therapists need knowledge and direction, not merely the exploration of countertransference and personal history (see Kernberg, 2010).

As I discuss in Chapter 5, in my supervision group at Rutgers, there have been a few times over the years when a student has, usually with a lot of hesitation, brought up a problem with a supervisor that turns out to reflect the supervisor's treating the clinician like a patient rather than a supervisee. Graduate students in clinical psychology tend to be very self-critical, and it may take them a long time to realize that there is something wrong with this approach. They typically try hard to cooperate with the supervisor, hoping there is some ultimate wisdom behind the requests for an uncomfortable degree of self-exposure. When they finally ask for feedback about their situation from the group, their classmates typically express dismay on their behalf, and their self-critical ruminations are finally interrupted and reframed.

But it typically takes a while before they themselves come to the realization that a polite objection, a firm renegotiation of boundaries, or even a change of supervisor might be in order. Part of their difficulty arriving at this position involves their dread of bringing complaints to a person who is treating them like a patient. A supervisor who tends to "interpret" instead of teach may also "interpret" a wish for change as if it were a psychodynamic issue rather than a reasonable criticism, with possible ramifications, admitting of practical resolutions. Thus, the student needs, with the group's help, to get to an internal place of feeling sturdy in the face of this possible response to legitimate grievances.

The problem here is that the contract between patient and therapist is significantly different from the contract between therapist and supervisor (see Moga & Cabaniss, 2014). Permission to critique a clinician's *work* is inherent in the supervisory contract, but permission to explore and interpret the therapist's *psychology* is not. As a supervisory relationship becomes more trusting, a student may begin to want to make connections between personal psychological patterns and clinical problems, but the initiative to go into that territory should come from the student. Mentors might mention aspects of the therapist's personality or behavior that they notice (e.g., "I get the sense that you are a particularly kind person, so the patient's sadistic side must be uncomfortable for you" or "I think I'm seeing a pattern of your avoiding the patient's criticism"), but making such observations is different from insisting that the student expose personal dynamics in the supervisory hour.

This kind of problem has not often been brought to my supervision group, but when it has come up, it is painful to witness the damage it has done to a student's self-esteem. When treated this way, without their consent to a high degree of intrusion into their mental life, student clinicians lose confidence, begin questioning what they know, and may infer that the supervisor has doubts about their competence or even their mental health. Having observed this situation several times, I have come down on the "teach" side of the teach-or-treat polarity (and even more on the side of trying to deconstruct the polarity itself, as teaching and treating are not pure or mutually exclusive options)—especially for clinicians in the early phases of their career at a time when they are most undone by insufficient support and excessive intrusion into areas of legitimate privacy.

I have arrived at this position also from my own experience as a therapist in training. Like most people in analytic supervision, when I started working with patients, I already had a therapist. What I needed from a seasoned colleague was not treatment but wisdom and advice about the clinical application of what I was learning: diagnostic reflections, suggestions for different ways to deal with clinical challenges, a theoretical and empirical understanding of various dilemmas, referrals to sources of knowledge about particular patients and problems, and so on. Early in my experience of supervision, even with nonintrusive supervisors, I felt skinless, that is, exposed to a painful degree. Any more undoing of my defenses would have overwhelmed me. I appreciated mentors who respected my boundaries, trusted my maturity, and tried to supplement my knowledge base and clinical judgment with digestible doses of nourishment.

On the other hand, I know of a few excellent supervisors with reputations for charging into the inner life of supervisees and evoking powerful emotional reactions. When trainees know that this is the supervisor's style, and when they have a choice about who supervises them, they can make an informed decision about whether to sign on for such in-depth, therapy-like supervision. My mentor Arthur Robbins took this approach; his teaching was inextricably linked to emotional expressiveness that felt therapeutic under his guidance. Except for my personal analysis, his was the most helpful training I ever had: It was genuinely therapeutic as well as educative. But I went into it explicitly giving permission for my dynamics to be examined, fully aware of Art's reputation for diving deep at a point when I was reasonably acquainted with my own unconscious. I had a sense also of his unique personality and could see that his intimate style reflected how he could most authentically be himself in the supervisory role. Thus, like most issues we tend to cast as either–or binaries, there are complexities that complicate the teach-versus-treat dichotomy. As Warren Wilner (2015) has observed, "supervision has a strong therapeutic dimension and therapy has a significant supervisory element" (p. 192).

Interestingly, an extensive naturalistic study conducted at the Columbia University Center for Psychoanalytic Training and Research (Cabaniss et al., 2001) found that institute candidates did not feel the degree of tension between teaching and treating that one would expect on the basis of the prominence of the issue in the literature. They thought, and the supervisors in the study agreed, that the role of supervisor is to teach, not treat, and yet they considered exploration of their own countertransference responses to be a legitimate part of teaching. Evidently, countertransference reactions have been sufficiently destigmatized in recent decades to have created a sea change in the general attitudes and expectations of supervisees. This is an important finding that highlights the value of doing research on the supervisory process.

Over the last century, attitudes about countertransference have evolved strikingly, from Freud's construing a therapist's emotional reactions to patients as evidence of "unresolved" personal dynamics resulting from an insufficiently thorough personal analysis to a later position (Racker, 1968) of construing affective arousal as ordinary and inevitable and mining it for meaning. The gradual understanding of intersubjective processes between therapist and patient, and between supervisor and supervisee, has slowly but radically reshaped the psychoanalytic landscape (see Berman, 2000; Jaffe, 2000). What was once considered private and even shameful is now regarded as both inevitable and valuable for understanding the clinical process. Even students who otherwise feel vulnerable seem to take for granted these days that they will have emotional reactions to their patients and that they will be expected to talk about them in supervision. I suspect that if supervisors ask about such responses in a tone that is collegial and respectful, and especially if they disclose without embarrassment what they are feeling in the parallel process, most supervisees would not experience queries about their countertransferences as unwelcome impingements.

To Teach Techniques or Foster Growth?

In the other recurring professional conversation, about whether supervision should be more about teaching skills or more about encouraging overall professional maturation, there is also no clear polarized

"winner." Because I have been concerned in recent decades that psychotherapy itself has been reframed by bureaucratic and financially biased
parties as a matter of mastering techniques rather than of nurturing
a healing relationship (McWilliams, 2005), I tilt toward the fostering
growth pole and the conceptualization of elements of supervision as
"processes" rather than reified interventions (cf. Bonovitz, 2010; Diener
& Mesrie, 2015). Despite my appreciation of the value of learning specific skills, I do not easily warm to the reduction of either psychotherapy
or supervision to expertise in certain "competencies."

What I find myself looking to help my supervisees expand includes
not practiced skills or techniques but mature attitudes: emotional honesty, respect for patients, open-minded curiosity, genuine empathy (as
opposed to rote sympathy), the capacity to mentalize even clients who
are difficult to like, an integration of their clinical knowledge with their
authentic personal style, an expansion into theoretical realms beyond
those they were trained in, humility, ethical sensitivity, a willingness to
admit to mistakes, and knowing where to go for help. These changes
occur not through pedagogy but in the context of a relationship that
moves organically toward more intimate and safer attachment.

Like "teach or treat," however, the question as it has been repeatedly posed is falsely dichotomous. Learning content cannot be separated
from internalizing a process through which the content is delivered.
Highly directive supervisors are not in control of whether their supervisees actually put into effect everything they are taught, and even students who want their supervisors to tell them the "right way" to treat
their clients have to assimilate what they learn through the style and
limits of their own personality. The affective elements of any educative experience make the acquisition of skills or information a complex
issue. Shame, fear, idealization, envy, identification, and other dynamics
are inextricably involved, and personal change (hopefully for the better)
is almost guaranteed in supervision, irrespective of how practical and
hands-on one's training is.

Once again, on the other hand (I may have run out of hands at
this point, but bear with me), despite my own allergy to framing psychotherapy as a collection of discrete techniques, it is clear to me that
to be a good-enough psychoanalytic therapist, one must master certain
skills, such as those delineated in the previous chapter. To insist that a
supervisory affiliation should be entirely exploratory, egalitarian, and
mutually influential, rather than accepting the reality that it is a "tilted"
(Greenacre, 1954) or "asymmetrical" (Aron, 1991) emotional relationship, in which a more experienced clinician has practical proficiencies to

teach the less experienced one, would be to ignore obvious inequalities of status and competence and to undermine the supervisee's legitimate right to learn what the supervisor knows. In addition, the reality that in many cases the professionally older colleague is responsible for evaluation and gatekeeping makes denial of the inherent relational hierarchy an indefensible attitude.

THE SUPERVISORY ALLIANCE

One of the challenges in conceptualizing supervision is that we all carry relatively unconscious metaphorical prototypes for our later life experiences that are based on our earlier experiences. As Ludwig Wittgenstein famously observed, the language in which we think determines what it is possible for us to imagine. The current tendencies in clinical psychology and psychiatry (social work and counseling have been somewhat different) to frame supervision as the teaching of a graduated skill set implicitly compares clinical maturation to artistic or athletic development. In these areas, an expert gives systematic, titrated advice about performance. Psychoanalytic supervision, especially as it has become more egalitarian and experiential over the decades, includes such a sensibility but also reflects an underlying model that is more developmental and mutually interpenetrating: The more experienced person struggles like a parent or caregiver to adapt to the maturational needs of each individual child; each supervisory dyad pursues a "good fit" (Escalona, 1968) and tries to grow together as a supervisory team (cf. Rosbrow, 1997).

Over the course of the evolution of psychotherapy, and not just psychodynamic therapy, there has been an increasing recognition of the determinative role of the therapeutic alliance in treatment outcome (e.g., Flückiger et al., 2012; Norcross & Wampold, 2011; Safran & Muran, 2003). In this century, researchers have demonstrated the importance of the relationship even in psychopharmacology: Patients who are given a placebo for their mental health problems *but who like their doctors* do measurably better than those who have a chillier relationship with their psychiatrists but are prescribed the actual medicine (Krupnik et al., 2006).

A parallel development that has emerged in the supervisory literature is an appreciation of the critical contribution of the "learning alliance" or "supervisory alliance" to effective supervision (Fleming & Benedek, 1966; Frijling-Schreuder, 1970; Gill, 2001; Teitelman, 1995;

Watkins, 2011). In the case of both the therapeutic and the supervisory alliance, an empirical literature attests to the primary role of interpersonal and emotional factors, although scientific studies on the therapeutic alliance remain much more numerous than investigations of the supervisory alliance. Much of this shift in emphasis is attributable to the realization, via both personal anecdote and research (e.g., Jaffe, 2001; Strømme, 2012), of how vulnerable supervisees feel when their work is examined in supervision (Slavin, 1998; Zicht, 2019). I address this vulnerability in the following chapter.

CONCLUDING COMMENTS

I have tried here to put psychoanalytic supervision in a historical context, starting with Sigmund Freud and progressing through different phases of its clinical and empirical evolution. I have raised questions originally posed by adherents of the Berlin and Budapest schools of psychoanalysis about the boundaries between psychotherapy and supervision, related that issue to other questions involving role responsibilities, and summarized and commented on two controversies (teaching versus treating and teaching skills versus supporting maturation) that have appeared recurrently in the clinical literature. Finally, I have commented on the evolving construct of the supervisory alliance, a critical conceptualization that I bring to bear on numerous issues in the subsequent chapters.

Chapter Three

■ ■ ■ ■

Psychological Vital Signs

EVALUATING PROGRESS IN TREATMENT

An overriding aim of supervision is the welfare of the supervisee's patients. Clinicians learning psychodynamic therapies thus need to learn how practitioners in the analytic tradition evaluate meaningful progress toward better mental health. This chapter covers 10 key areas in which the psychological vital signs of change and growth may occur. Supervisors tend naturally to keep their eye on these areas, and supervisees need to learn to monitor them on their own. These vital signs differ substantially from the symptom-reduction criteria most researchers use to evaluate manualized short-term treatments. Although analytic therapies have always aimed at reducing troubling symptoms (e.g., states of mind such as anxiety and depression), even short-term psychodynamic models of care typically pursue more general goals. Recent empirical work (e.g., De Smet et al., 2020) suggests that patients also regard symptom reduction as secondary to broader outcomes, such as feeling more empowered and finding more balance.

A brief distinction between clinical and research objectives is in order here. In investigations into comparative treatment outcomes, scientists must stipulate changes that their studies will accept as evidence of progress. The most practical criteria involve improvement in DSM-related symptoms that can be measured by validated, reliable instruments. In clinical practice, in contrast, patient and therapist identify together the goals toward which they will work. Many clients seek psychotherapy for concerns that do not map well onto DSM categories: They want to improve overall life satisfaction, make critical personal decisions, break out of problematic relational patterns, feel internally more confident, begin looking seriously at their substance use, grieve a painful loss, come out as gay or trans, face a developmental crisis, be a better parent, and so on.

Most DSM diagnostic categories are not really "illnesses" but symptoms of some underlying issue: Consciously or unconsciously, we feel anxious or depressed *about* something. During the course of an effective therapy, symptoms may wax and wane as patients work on more fundamental goals, such as increased life satisfaction and the prevention of future psychopathology. A focus on symptom reduction is often useful, but sometimes it can distract from these overall therapeutic aims. Supervisees should be prepared to accept the fact that in an ambitious treatment, symptoms may temporarily worsen rather than consistently abate.

For example, individuals taking the risk of behaving in more adaptive but unfamiliar ways will likely feel increased anxiety; those who, after a long period of denial and somatization, begin to grieve a terrible loss may score temporarily as more depressed on the Beck Depression Inventory even though their mourning will be ultimately therapeutic. Sometimes, patients complain that they are progressing too slowly when there is evidence that unconsciously they are frightened that changes are happening too fast for them to assimilate. Sometimes, after they take some qualitative steps toward greater health, they regress into old patterns for a while. Supervisees need to know that this backsliding does not mean that the progress was illusory.

As Jonathan Shedler has persuasively argued (2019), most DSM "disorders" are more like a skin rash, fever, or limp than a medical illness. They signal that something is wrong in the overall psychological system. Although medicine does not organize *physical* problems under symptom categories (e.g., "skin rash disorders," "fever disorders," "limp disorders"), psychiatry, for a host of intersecting reasons, has opted to do so, and other powerful interests have reinforced this choice. Pharmaceutical corporations are fond of symptom-defined categories because they can market drugs that target those symptoms. Third-party payers like them because alleviating symptoms is faster and cheaper than healing what gave rise to them. Many academicians like them because they are easier to measure than other psychological changes, and they expedite the completion of the kinds of studies that are easy to accumulate on one's publication record. Some patients and their families like them because being afflicted with a DSM "disorder" may seem less vilifying of the self and others than thinking about their difficulties in more probing ways.

The fact that diagnosing based on categorical symptom syndromes is attractive to certain interested parties does not make such unidimensional labels a reasonable or scientific way to conceptualize human psychological suffering. Nor does it privilege them for devising treatment plans. Psychodynamic clinicians, whose focus has always been on the meaning and function of symptoms, tend to see the claims of the previous two sentences as self-evident. But they are also supported by research. Tom Insel, former director of the National Institute for Mental Health, has independently reached similar conclusions (Insel & Gogtay, 2014), as have many researchers in psychopathology (e.g., Sharp et al., 2015; Weinberger & Stoycheva, 2020).

Nevertheless, DSM categories still dominate our current terminology, and beginning supervisees are usually accustomed to speaking in that language. I therefore want to specify some psychological ideals that are more centrally the concern of psychodynamic therapy than attention to the criteria that define DSM disorders. Nonpsychoanalytic therapists have not ignored these areas, but they have less consistently foregrounded them in their clinical writing. An exception is the substantial empirically based literature on positive psychology (e.g., Lopez, Pedrotti, & Snyder, 2018), but this movement has tended to highlight and prioritize the goal of personal happiness (e.g., Seligman, 2004). Psychoanalytic therapists certainly appreciate states of happiness, and we like our patients to be happy, but we are careful not to endorse hypomanic solutions to life's problems, and we tend to emphasize more strongly the overall mental health value of capacities to tolerate grief, shame, guilt, and other negative affect states.

In what follows, I focus primarily on the supervision of beginning therapists, as clinicians with more experience tend to be already familiar with monitoring these vital signs. Where I know of parallel terms for specific capacities that have been used by cognitive-behavioral psychology, general humanistic psychology, or the positive psychology movement, I mention them. A somewhat differently organized and more comprehensive and detailed list of these vital signs can be found in the "Profile of Mental Functioning" for each age range covered in the second edition of the *Psychodynamic Diagnostic Manual (PDM-2)* (Lingiardi & McWilliams, 2017). In this organization of psychological vital signs, I rather arbitrarily group overall mental health criteria under 10 headings, focusing on the implications of each one for psychoanalytic supervision.

SAFETY AND INCREASED ATTACHMENT SECURITY

Extensive research on attachment attests to the critical role of basic relational security in overall mental health (Cassidy & Shaver, 2016). Securely attached children are better off in virtually every measurable way, and the inverse is true as well: There is a powerful relationship between the *absence* of emotional safety and the severity of psychopathology (e.g., Luyten, Vliegen, Van Houdenhove, & Blatt, 2008). The first job of any therapist with any patient is to create a relationship that feels as safe as possible. The internalization of such a relationship is a core element, probably *the* core element, in most psychological healing (American Psychological Association, 2012; Norcross & Wampold, 2019).

Supervisees may be familiar with one or more terms for psychological security. Probably the best known is Erikson's (1950) positing "basic trust" as the primary developmental concern. In Maslow's hierarchy of needs (1943), safety is right above the physiological requirements for survival. Recent students of psychology tend to be familiar with concepts of "secure attachment" and "safe harbor" coined by John Bowlby (1969, 1973) and then elaborated in decades of research by his students (e.g., Ainsworth & Bell, 1970; see Beebe & Lachmann, 2014; Eagle, 2013). The analytic literature also includes Sullivan's concept of "ontological security" (1953), Eigen's "area of faith" (1981), and Fonagy's more contemporary, research-derived emphasis on "epistemic trust" (Allison & Fonagy, 2016; Bateman & Fonagy, 2013). Cognitive-behavioral psychologists attend to similar issues when they identify and address "safety behaviors" (e.g., Helbig-Lang & Petermann, 2010). Psychotherapy can create "earned attachment" (see Solye & Strathearn, 2017); in long-term treatment, clinicians can foster a shift from a less to a more secure attachment style (Mikulincer & Shaver, 2016). But even in short-term work, it is critical to keep one's eye on the issue of basic relational safety.

Supervisors may need to remind supervisees that just because they are trustworthy and well intentioned, their patients may not see them that way. If a person's earliest experience with authorities is replete with neglect and betrayal, trust in another's benevolence has no emotional foundation. We all know intuitively how far the plea "Trust me!" goes when there is not yet credible evidence for someone's trustworthiness. But it is hard on trainees to learn that when they invite clients to trust them, their own realistic trustworthiness is grossly insufficient to reassure a skeptical patient. It tends to surprise and disappoint beginners that trust building will take a long time; it can comfort them to learn that even experienced clinicians can be shocked when, after years of devoted care, a patient seizes on some perceived misattunement as "proof" of the therapist's basic unreliability.

Before trying to "do therapy," the clinician may need to find practical ways to increase a patient's sense of safety. Beyond having been urged to be empathic and respectful of clients' subjective experiences, newer therapists are unlikely to have had classroom training in dealing with patients who see them as a threat. This territory covers both the therapeutic setting (e.g., asking if a paranoid patient wants to sit nearer to the office door) and the clinician's openness to hearing without defensiveness about fears that the therapist is dangerous. Seasoned practitioners know that such anxieties take multiple and sometimes surprising forms. For example, I once worked with a psychoanalytically sophisticated man who told me that my warmth was intolerable to him, as it invited an emotional exposure and regression that he was afraid would leave him in pieces. "You're not going to pull any of that Carl Rogers shit on me, are you?!" he demanded. Some patients—especially those who are more seriously disturbed—do not want a therapist penetrating and influencing their mind, and they feel profoundly unsafe when they sense that such an invasion has happened.

It is sometimes a new idea to supervisees, especially those trained in academic programs that emphasize measurable, testable criteria, that the evidence of significant change may appear more clearly in a patient's "asides" or seemingly incidental remarks than in the findings of assessment instruments; for example, the casual mention by a man with formerly severe separation anxiety that he recently enjoyed a weekend alone. Michael Garrett (2019) treated a woman with the delusional belief that she smelled bad; she heard the voices of "crack addicts" in the neighboring apartment regularly lamenting her odor. One day after several weeks of treatment, she informed him that there was a new crack addict in the building, one who said she did not smell. She was still hallucinating, but she had internalized something positive. Sometimes clients seem unaware of the profound implications of a passing comment; at other times, they clearly know that something important has happened.

I remember in this context a woman with disabling paranoid anxieties who came into my office after about a year and a half of our working together, looking a bit shaken. As she approached her usual chair, she mused, "A strange thing happened on my way here." Expecting her to talk about something she had witnessed on the way to my office, I asked her what she was referring to. She replied, "I found myself thinking, 'You're going to feel better after you talk to Nancy about this.' And

I have never felt that way toward anyone in my life!" For a while after that, as is so typical of the back-and-forth-ness of recovery, she became more paranoid, evidently because it terrified her to find herself expecting help from another human being. But that paranoid episode turned out to be a temporary regression from an overall trend toward a greater sense of safety.

Needless to say, a therapist who experiences a benign atmosphere in supervision will be better at making patients feel safe than one who feels constantly vulnerable and anxious, or, for that matter, one who intuits excessive anxiety in the supervisor (Sherman, 2015). In addition to the importance of maximizing a sense of security in the supervisory relationship (Slavin, 1998; Zicht, 2019), the main implication for supervisors regarding the goal of increased relationship security involves helping supervisees to modify their more natural reaction to being distrusted, which is to try to demonstrate their trustworthiness. Instead, they have to cultivate comfort with patients' lack of trust. Helping them to help their clients express their misgivings and suspicions, and to tolerate their own painful affects when they succeed in this effort, offers a more reliable route to interpersonal safety than efforts to demonstrate goodness. Supervisees who cannot tolerate their patients' hostility and wariness risk acting defensively when they should be welcoming all aspects of the client's subjectivity into the relationship.

SELF- AND OBJECT CONSTANCY

Building self- and object constancy is a second overarching focus of psychodynamic work. A key part of mental wellness is the capacity to see the self and others as complex and generally consistent individuals, with both good and bad aspects, who are not subject to abrupt and catastrophic transformation. Efforts to overcome "splitting" (Kernberg, 1975; Klein, 1946) have been central to the psychoanalytic idea of therapeutic progress; supervisees familiar with dialectical behavior therapy (DBT) may rightly note its similarity to Marsha Linehan's (1993) emphasis on developing dialectical rather than either–or thinking.

Freud (1920) was fascinated by the psychological meaning of infant delight in games like peek-a-boo. He watched his grandson repeatedly moving an object in and out of his visual field and proclaiming "Fort!" ("Here!") and then "Da!" ("There!") as the boy mastered the knowledge that objects continue to exist even when out of sight. In appreciation of the work of his colleague Jean Piaget (1923/2011), the great cognitive psychologist who had been analyzed by Sabina Spielrein, scholars have called this achievement "object permanence." The more relational notion of "object constancy," the sense that a human love object remains emotionally connected even when physically absent, and also can be trusted not to morph into a persecutor, was first elaborated by Melanie Klein (1946). Although Klein's writing is difficult reading, I have found that supervisees appreciate a short explication of her ideas, especially her concepts of the paranoid–schizoid and the depressive positions, respectively.

Supervisees need to understand their own normal fluctuation between the paranoid–schizoid state, in which we see the self and others in all-good or all-bad terms, and the depressive position that affords a sense of continuity and allows others to be emotionally three-dimensional. In the depressive position, we recognize the separate subjectivity of the other, and we appreciate that good and bad coexist in both the self and others. Later terms for psychological constancy include "identity integration" (Erikson, 1968) (and its opposite, "identity diffusion" [Kernberg, 1984]) and also "self-cohesion" (and its opposite, "self-fragmentation" [Kohut, 1971]). Sullivan's (1953) notion of "malevolent transformation" of a good other into a mean-spirited, treacherous antagonist captures the same phenomenon: absence of the continuity that Winnicott (1963) called "going on being."

Supervisees need to learn to distinguish between patients who have a reliable sense of self-continuity and the continuity of others, who can go back and forth between the paranoid–schizoid and depressive positions, from those who live in a consistently frightening paranoid–schizoid world where anything can happen at any time, where alien states of mind can suddenly take over, and where the self and others are dangerously subject to malevolent transformation. Supervisees need to distinguish between changes of emotional valence and changes of self-state; that is, they need to understand something about dissociative experiences in which continuity with memory, with feelings, with one's body, with knowledge, and with one's basic sense of self disappears (see Howell, 2020).

In the absence of attention to this area, newer therapists tend to assume that because they themselves may feel a sense of continuity in time and space, their patients do as well. They may misunderstand sudden changes in the client's self-state as simply shifts of mood. They may need guidance in figuring out how to help the person develop some sense of what Bromberg (1998) called "standing in the spaces" between different states of mind. The evolution of this capacity is far more important than the temporary relief of painful affects. Appreciation of its absence in one's patient has profound, wide-ranging implications that supervisors can helpfully spell out.

Let me illustrate with attention to the special problem of continuity for patients with backgrounds of trauma. With so much pressure these days to deliver brief treatments, it is particularly important for supervisors to emphasize that for posttraumatic patients, the slower you go, the faster you get there. New therapists will be hearing or will have heard the opposite message for some time, on the basis of studies with patients who are on average considerably healthier than the ones who seek their help. For clients with complex trauma and sexual abuse histories, the sense that someone is trying to rush them can trigger feelings about prior subjugations to the agendas of others. At best, moving too fast will stymie such patients; at worst, it can retraumatize them. Experts in trauma and dissociation have consistently made this point (e.g., Chefetz, 2015).

Beginning clinicians may themselves need to be slowed down when survivors of complex trauma express impatience with therapy and seem to need more frequent sessions, or when they explicitly ask for such an accommodation. The clinician's natural response may be to agree to more appointments, since most of us who are attracted to psychoanalytic work value the depth that greater frequency can promote. But posttraumatic patients, given their background of being used and hurt by prior authorities, may have severe unconscious terror about entering a more intense attachment. Increased frequency may provoke regressive suffering rather than comfort and security. Supervisors may have to explain that although frequency is a good thing in general, it can dysregulate clients with trauma histories. A sense of continuity is unlikely to evolve in the context of one crisis after another.

One suggestion I sometimes give to supervisees in this situation involves first interpreting the patient's unconscious fears of intimacy (e.g., "I appreciate that you want to meet more frequently, but at the same time, I suspect that you have a coexisting and powerful unconscious fear of greater closeness that we need to respect"). I may go on to suggest, "I'm open to working with you three times a week once I can see that you're doing pretty well with twice. If you can go for a couple of months without _____ [dissociating, attempting suicide, binge drinking, acting out sexually, or whatever has been the patient's tendency], let's consider that together." This makes a deeper connection conditional on the patient's getting better rather than worse, avoids inciting or rewarding regression, and reassures clients that the therapist is not going to dive into their most painful self-states at a psychologically intolerable pace. I might frame the therapist's (and the supervisor's) role in this situation in terms of Winnicott's concept of "holding" or Bion's (1962) concept of "containment."

This is only one example how a supervisor keeps an eye on the clinician's efforts to foster self- and object constancy. Another supervisory activity that fosters this goal is calling attention to any instances of the therapist's own normal splitting, or that of the supervisor. For example, it is natural, especially for newer clinicians, to see their patients positively while viewing the patient's current or former caregivers as evil. It takes a leap of empathy to resist framing the patient as the good one and the parent as a monster and to avoid interventions that split. Supervisors need to encourage therapists to offer comments like, "Wow. That's a terrible mistake your mother made. Do you think she was under the misunderstanding that it would be good for you? What do you know about her own history that could account for this disastrous behavior?"

Similarly, when a supervisee makes one authority the good one and another the bad one, or buys into the patient's split between the therapist and a group leader, couple's counselor, or physician, the splitting process can be identified and problematized. Sometimes a consultation with the other party may be called for (with appropriate permission) so that any disagreements in formulation and direction of treatment can be aired and resolved. Whether or not the student is right about who is better and worse overall, the situation needs to be viewed in context and understood in more complex terms. I find it useful to confess to supervisees my own splitting reactions, while trying simultaneously to exemplify the obligation to have a less binary attitude—for example, "I find myself absolutely hating this father! But we need to remember that we're hearing this story via the client's one-dimensional experience of him, and part of what we hope to do eventually is give her a more nuanced understanding of the man and his history and possible dynamics."

SENSE OF AGENCY (AUTONOMY, SELF-EFFICACY)

Psychoanalytic clinical literature evidences consistent concern for supporting and increasing each patient's sense of agency. Some of the snarkier caricatures of psychodynamic technique lampoon our efforts to pursue this goal ("What do *you* think about this?"; "What do *you* see as the options here?"; "What are *your* associations to the dream?"). Analytic practitioners do tend to be reluctant to give advice. Following someone else's direction, even when that person's advice is good, does not increase patients' confidence about their own problem-solving capacities. In addition, advice giving tends to support one side of a client's internal conflict rather than making the person's ambivalence available for consideration. Because some of their prior academic mentors will have characterized the psychoanalytic resistance to taking an authoritative position as laziness or knee-jerk rule following, supervisors should be prepared both to defend the values that underlie the stereotypes and to identify areas in which a client's autonomy can be supported with less robotic comments.

Let me ground the concept of agency in psychoanalytic developmental theory, with which some trainees may have been acquainted as students, but which they now need to connect to real-life clinical material. Jung's (1921) concept of "individuation" was an early focus on the goal of an agentic self. Erikson (1950) referred to this aspect of mental health as "autonomy" (a term with Greek roots suggesting "self-governance"), which later matures into a sense of "initiative." A closely related, more recent term is "self-efficacy" (e.g., Frank, 2001). Most analytic writers call the feeling that one can have an impact on one's environment and future a "sense of agency." In talking with clients about it, we use expressions like "finding your voice," "negotiating on your own behalf," or "stopping to think before complying." Good psychotherapy creates the conditions for its own expiration because the patient will no longer need the therapist. As Winnicott (1968) noted, "We all hope our patients will finish with us and forget us, and that they will find living itself to be the therapy that makes sense" (p. 712).

The concept of autonomy reflects a Western bias in the direction of individualism. When supervisees work with patients from more collectivist cultures, they should be helped to adapt the ideal of a sense of agency to those contexts. When I have talked about agency to colleagues in Turkey, the Far East, and communitarian subcultures in North America, they tell me that despite their culture's putting less emphasis on individual freedom, they do not lack the goal of living an agentic life. A Chinese therapist explained, "We think of maturation in terms of increasing obligations to care for others. But we can tell the difference between people who feel they have no choice in how to do so and those who can find their own way to carry out their commitments."

Supervisees need to be oriented toward inferring each patient's degree of felt power to influence events. Many people begin treatment feeling that things just "happen to" them. The absence of a sense of agency is inferable when the therapist has asked a question such as, "Were you feeling sexual desire when you agreed to give oral sex to that guy?" and meets a blank stare or a response like "I don't know. It seemed like the thing to do at the time." Patients who give such answers are often the same ones who wait passively for the therapist to tell them what to do, a stance that can flummox clinicians learning analytic therapy, who know that it does not involve following a set of instructions but do not easily find their own sense of agency in the face of this nonparticipation. Psychodynamic therapists want clients to feel increasing power to influence their own lives, to find their own tools, to question any sense they carry around of being inevitably victimized, controlled by others, or helplessly vulnerable to random trauma.

Individuals who seek treatment may, understandably, just want the pain to stop. They may view clinicians as authorities who will simply fix their feelings, or fix their partner or boss or parent. They may have been told that there are active strategies that therapists can implement. New therapists feel acute pressure to perform such magic, especially if their training has emphasized evidence-based techniques or medication that, in terms of statistical averages, can reduce immediate pain. But patients who are helped to find the confidence that *they* can change what is making them unhappy get something much more valuable than temporary relief from a toxic mental state. We know that therapy can repair what Panksepp (1998) has called the SEEKING system (which is largely dopamine driven) and strengthen the ability of the prefrontal cortex (which controls executive function) to manage urgent messages from the amygdala (Buchheim et al., 2012).

There are some patients—for example, those suffering psychotic conditions—whose sense of agency lies in giving the therapist material on which the therapist can act. For example, a delusional man who is tortured by insomnia can feel a minimal sense of agency in persuading a psychiatrist to prescribe a sleep aid. And sometimes showing that one has gotten the message and can do something is a good first step in building the therapeutic alliance and modeling agency. But in general, clinicians need supervisory support to avoid falling into the role of fixer, which tends to be either ineffective in changing behavior or, when effective in the short run, reinforces the conviction that all the person has to do in life is find an authority whose directions can be followed.

Supervisees also need help not to fall into the complementary role of helpless bystander. Between trying to fix things for patients and passively witnessing their misery there are usually several options to explore in supervision. Clinicians working with nonagentic clients may need first to vent their frustration in supervision: They typically find themselves working harder than the patient. Many supervisors have told their students that if they are doing more than half the heavy lifting, they should back off and look with the client at what is going on. Clinicians often do not know how to achieve this balance and need assistance in turning countertransference futility into creative problem solving. Supervisors of therapists treating passive, helpless patients thus need to help them recover their own sense of efficacy.

One way to do so is to role-play several alternative solutions. Identifying options together, and having the therapist choose the most promising approach may help restore the clinician's sense of inner-directedness. A supervisee portraying the patient will likely enjoy frustrating the supervisor, and with the humor that results, a grimly static situation can become more playful. Options might include, for example, (1) saying very little until the patient fills the silent space; (2) expressing one's own dilemma (e.g., "I'm not sure how to help you here. You came to me to find your own voice, but I feel a degree of pressure from you to impose *my* voice on your predicament. When I do that, I undermine your capacity to find your own way, but when I don't do it, you seem very unhappy"); (3) asking what is going on in the patient's somatic experience (e.g., "What are you feeling physically right now, and where in your body is the feeling located?"); (4) commenting on the repetition of an old relational pattern (e.g., "It seems like you and I are being cast into roles that parallel the emotional themes of your childhood, as if the only way to experience our work is that one of us is a demanding parent and the other a sullen child"). And so on. Even if none of these strategies work very well, the process of considering them may give the supervisee some recovery of a feeling of agency and an appreciation of how vital that capacity is.

REALISTIC AND RELIABLE SELF-ESTEEM (HEALTHY NARCISSISM)

Issues of self-esteem are central to overall mental health. The more realistically based and stable is our self-regard, the more likely we are to avoid developing disorders of personality, addiction, or behavior, and to be protected from psychotic deterioration. A focus on self-esteem has always been part of psychoanalytic practice and has expanded as we have seen more problems in this area in recent decades. The earliest analysts were trying to help people whose self-esteem suffered from unreasonably oppressive standards, such as demands on women not to feel sexual desire until "awakened" by a husband or pressures on men to adopt an extreme code of honor. These early psychoanalytic patients tended to suffer from severe and irrational guilt and viewed their lives in terms of unending duties and obligations, a condition that Karen Horney (1950) later popularized as "the tyranny of the shoulds."

Later in the 20th century, the kinds of self-esteem problems for which patients sought help shifted from such complaints (often described as involving a "harsh superego") toward a sense of inner emptiness and confusion about core values. The extensive literature on self-esteem is often misunderstood in popular culture, in which strategies to improve it, such as giving high grades to everyone, irrespective of the quality of the work, may be shallow, "feel-good" measures that are often counter-productive to the development of a sense of self-worth based on honest self-examination (see Battan, 1983; Lasch, 1978).

The concept of self-esteem that emerges from the writings of influential 20th-century psychotherapists (e.g., Rank, Adler, Rogers, Maslow, Murray, Allport, and Kohut) denotes a slowly maturing and eventually stable property of personality. Self-esteem that is *realistic* reflects reasonable (i.e., neither perfectionistic nor falsely inflated) criteria for self-evaluation. Self-esteem that is *reliable* protects against being devastated by criticism or manipulated by adulation. It allows us to evaluate negative feedback without collapsing internally and positive feedback without being seduced by flattery. Healthy self-esteem comes from internalizing caregivers' nonshaming attitudes toward our authentic feelings, thoughts, and behaviors. If parental standards are reasonable, we feel a sense of self-approval when we measure up, and we try to improve if we fall short. Unreasonable standards, conveyed by sadistic criticism or empty praise, have pathologically depressive or narcissistic consequences. Neglect of all standards causes children to take their yardstick from cultural icons, which may (think superheroes, vapid celebrities, commercial advertising), lead to perverse and unachievable aspirations.

Individuals with adequate self-esteem are levelheaded about their limitations and failings as well as their strengths. Because their self-image embraces states of inevitable fault and need, they can apologize when they hurt others and express gratitude when they are helped. They can make their needs explicit rather than expecting others to divine what they want and grant their wishes without their having to ask. They can say how they feel and talk in "I-statements" rather than deflecting blame. They can bear being deeply known and consequently can enjoy genuine emotional intimacy. Supervisees can usefully alert their mentees to the question of whether or not the patient can genuinely apologize, show gratitude, and ask for what is needed rather than simply complain.

Patients with solid self-esteem are easy to help, as are supervisees with the same advantage. But therapeutic practice is hard on the self-esteem of even a confident clinician.

A key challenge for supervisors attempting to help their mentees to encourage clients toward realistic, reliable self-esteem is that beginners often try to repair self-devaluation or compensatory self-inflation by commenting to patients on their good qualities, giving the equivalent of pep talks. As seasoned therapists know, this approach tends to backfire: Patients with poor self-esteem may conclude from positive feedback that the therapist does not really know them and has been duped into thinking they are worthy; patients with defensively inflated self-esteem may feel the therapist is wasting their time belaboring the obvious. Supervisors must break the news gently to their supervisees that their well-intentioned efforts may be intensifying depression or reinforcing pathological narcissism. Then they should offer better ways to support realistic and reliable self-esteem, such as challenging a critical superego rather than trying to prop up a damaged ego (see McWilliams, 2011, chapter 11) or exploring low self-regard or high entitlement without automatically trying to "fix" it.

In Chapter 4, I address the supervisor's support for the supervisee's self-esteem in greater depth, emphasizing tactful but honest feedback and efforts to provide enough emotional safety that the supervisee can disclose mistakes and failures without undue anxiety. In parallel, supervisees need to learn from their mentors how to invite their patients to disclose the ugliest aspects of themselves so that they can feel fully seen and accepted despite their limitations, transgressions, and vulnerabilities.

RESILIENCE, FLEXIBILITY, AND AFFECT REGULATION (EGO STRENGTH)

There is a long history in psychodynamic scholarship of evaluating "ego strength" (e.g., Bellak, Hurvich, & Gediman, 1973), the capacity to respond adaptively even under significant stress. The more contemporary term is "resilience" (e.g., Ginsberg, 2014), a conceptualization that has been extensively studied by researchers, especially those in the positive psychology movement. There continues to be uncertainty among scientists, however, about why some children seem undone by adverse emotional experiences, while others seem psychologically strengthened by them. Clinically, this question is seldom our focus; we tend to see people who are undone by stress and trauma, and we try to help them become emotionally stronger.

Resilience during and after adversity requires the capacities to bear strong feelings ("affect tolerance"), modulate them ("affective processing" or "affect regulation"), and govern their expression so that they lead to adaptive rather than destructive outcomes. In general, while cognitive-behavioral therapists have tended to emphasize the *control* of emotions that may incite bad behavior (as in "anger management"), psychodynamic clinicians have tended to focus on understanding, accepting, and reducing toxic affect states (e.g., shame, envy, despair) that may underlie emotional dysregulation and acting out (e.g., Gilligan, 1996). Psychoanalytic therapists typically urge patients to "put it into words" or "feel your feelings" when they are reeling from current stresses and the activation of traumatic histories.

Helping supervisees tolerate patients' extreme or atypical emotional reactions is a core part of psychoanalytic supervision. Overwhelming states of mind are sometimes wordless, announcing themselves in silent rage and pain that are unmistakable in body language and facial affect, but may be unavailable to the patient's conscious mind, either because of defenses like denial and dissociation or because such feelings are unformulated (see Stern, 1997, 2009). Alexithymic clients (those who lack words for affect) (Sifneos, 1973) tend to be especially difficult for newer psychoanalytic therapists (Taylor & Bagby, 2013). Neuroimaging studies of alexithymia (e.g., Craig, 2009) show that the brains of people who lack words for affect are genuinely not processing the emotions that seem so obvious to witnesses of their behavior. Being patient with alexithymic clients is not easy; clinicians need supportive supervision to hang in with them as they learn to formulate their inchoate somatic experience in the language of emotion (Stern, 1997, 2009).

In working with other clients, therapists may be deluged with uninhibited hate-filled, prejudicial, or despairing language for which their prior education has not prepared them. Despite having encouraged their clients to "say everything," it is hard for them not to be defensive—to become paralyzed, immersed in critical self-scrutiny, or provoked into explaining themselves or engaging in essentially political arguments—in the face of clients' personal attacks. Supervision is vital in helping therapists tolerate being treated in ways that the term "negative transference" doesn't even begin to capture. Increasing the therapist's resilience is the best path to increasing that of the patient.

The main way that analytic therapy builds ego strength is by creating a secure relational base, a "holding environment" (Winnicott, 1965) into which the patient slowly relaxes. Eventually, the internalized therapist's voice calms affective storms and orients the person toward possible ways of coping. But clients may need specific help while that slow internalization is happening. In nonpsychoanalytic treatments, they are often taught strategies for affect regulation (e.g., square breathing, brainspotting, somatic experiencing, or DBT skills for handling emotional overwhelm). Some analytic supervisors teach supervisees how to integrate such techniques into psychodynamic therapies or advise them to suggest relevant books and videos to patients. Others teach them mindfulness, meditation, and breathing processes that help manage dysregulated affect. Others integrate eye movement desensitization and reprocessing (EMDR) into psychoanalytic work. Mentors with training in such strategies can pass them along, or support their use in supervisees who already know them, without undermining the overall analytic process.

Critical to resilience is the use of defenses and coping skills that are both mature and flexible. In *Psychoanalytic Diagnosis* (McWilliams, 2011), I reviewed the most common primitive and higher-order defenses, respectively, and noted the developmental achievement of using sublimation and humor to cope with stress. Supervisors can teach clinicians to keep their eye on opportunities to help patients manage feelings with more adaptive defenses. For example, when suffering intense shame or envy, clients can learn to identify with aspects of the other rather than resorting to instant devaluation or self-attack. Eventually, they can be helped to regard their reactivity with self-compassion and humor and learn to take pride in expanding their range of responses beyond their typical defense, whether it is denial, avoidance, dissociation, splitting, or another automatic strategy to reduce mental pain. Because this kind of growth can take years, mentors can help clinicians to note evidence of patients' small steps in the direction of defensive maturity and flexibility.

REFLECTIVE FUNCTION (INSIGHT) AND MENTALIZATION

Psychodynamic therapists have always valued insight. Freud framed self-understanding as a cause of therapeutic change, and sometimes it is. But it can also be a *consequence* of the changes that happen in good treatment (Messer & McWilliams, 2006), and in analytic therapy it is a goal in itself, not just a means to an end. A capacity to reflect on the self (the "observing ego" of Richard Sterba, 1934, or the "reflective function" of Fonagy and Target, 1996) has long been clinically and empirically associated with a good outcome. When patients lack an introspective capacity, helping them develop it is a primary therapeutic aim. In recent analytic literature, there has been an emphasis not only on insight into the self, but also on insight into others, a faculty that philosophers call "theory of mind." The capacity to appreciate the separate subjectivities of other people has been highlighted in concepts such as Klein's (1946) "depressive position," Benjamin's "recognition" (2017), Fonagy's (e.g., Fonagy & Target, 1996) "mentalization," and Jurist's (2018) "mentalized affectivity." It is at the heart of Martin Buber's (1937) "I–Thou relationships."

In the absence of the capacity to reflect and mentalize, we project our own dynamics and motives into other people. The father of a 9-month-old baby once told me, "That kid knows just how to push my buttons!" Because he could not imagine the mental state of an infant, he experienced his child self-referentially, taking the baby's distress personally. Experienced psychodynamic clinicians help supervisees to notice instances of patients' failure to mentalize, and they work to help them foster that capacity. Evidence for a problem in mentalizing often is presented via transference experiences. When a therapist's words hurt their feelings, patients who cannot imagine the clinician's separate subjectivity may feel persecuted and be unable to see that the therapist is trying to be helpful. They may insist instead that "You're trying to hurt me" or even "You *like* to hurt me!"

Therapists themselves may, of course, be deficient in mentalization, as all of us are to some degree. They may need supervisory help to avoid relying on what Kleinians call "projection of intent." They may, for example, readily conclude that the way a patient's behavior makes them feel is what the patient *intends* for them to feel (e.g., "She dresses revealingly, so she must have sexual designs on me," or "It irritates me that this guy puts his coat on my chair, so it must be a hostile act"). It is a vital part of the supervisory role to encourage clinicians to consider other motivational possibilities than those based on their own projections. Reflective function and a capacity to mentalize others can continue to mature throughout life. Supervision often sets in motion or accelerates this growth process.

COMFORT IN BOTH COMMUNALITY AND INDIVIDUALITY

Psychological health requires both the capacity to engage collaboratively with other people and the capacity to stand alone and represent one's personal interests. Cultures vary in their emphases on communality versus individualism: As I noted in the section on agency, many Asian civilizations and tribal cultures have a primary focus on collectivity, whereas most Western postindustrial societies stress individuality (Jones, 2004). My experience in collaborating with therapists in other cultures again suggests that across different communities, there are consensual (often tacit) criteria for judging when someone is deficient in one of these capacities, in whatever way a given society defines it.

In Western diagnostic conventions, many conditions that are seen as inherently pathological have a heavy tilt toward the pole of either individuality or communality at the expense of capacities at the other end of that polarity. For example, overly dependent people need therapeutic help to feel comfortable resisting pressure from others, speaking their minds, and sometimes giving their own needs priority over others' wishes. Conversely, psychopathically manipulative people need a focus on developing concern for others rather than being "out for Number One" to a destructive extent.

Sidney Blatt (e.g., 2008) devoted several decades to studying this dimension of human psychology, beginning with trying to understand the difference between the inner experience of the depressed person who feels subjectively empty, lonely, needy, and shameful (the "anaclitic" type of depression) and the person with identical symptoms who feels internally bad and guilty (the "introjective" type). Supervisors can greatly increase supervisees' clinical effectiveness by helping them distinguish which version of depression predominates in their patient and noting the clinical implications of that distinction (Auerbach, 2019; Lingiardi, McWilliams, & Muzi, 2017).

Blatt eventually observed that many other psychologies, not just depressive states, can be depicted in terms of where one lies on the spectrum that he eventually construed as "self-in-relation versus self-definition." In both editions of the *Psychodynamic Diagnostic Manual* (Lingiardi & McWilliams, 2017; PDM Task Force, 2006), we addressed some implications of Blatt's polarity for personality types and the treatment of personality pathology. Interestingly, Blatt's research did not show that people who test as the psychologically healthiest occupy a midpoint between these poles. Instead, they are robust on both ends. That is, overall mental wellness involves a capacity to stand alone and *also* to surrender oneself to something greater (cf. Ghent, 1990) and to move fluidly between individual and communal concerns, experiencing comfort in both places.

Supervisors may be more sensitive to this polarity than some new therapists are, despite the fact that in general, educated younger people are more culturally sensitive than older professionals, especially those of us who are white and privileged. It is part of the supervisory role to be sure that a clinician is not, for example, pathologizing a patient from a culture in which the polarity is understood differently from the culture or subculture in which the therapist grew up. Cultural differences are often important to state out loud and to observe with interest rather than criticism.

When I was teaching in China a few years ago, a group of female therapists asked me an interesting question: How can we help our depressed grandmothers? They went on to explain that their grand-mothers had grown up at a time when women were valued for their chastity and were expected to be obedient to men: first to their fathers, then to their husbands, then to their sons. These clinicians had come of age two generations later, when female sexuality was more accepted in China and when occupational choice and greater autonomy had become available to many women. They wondered whether their grandmothers felt envy toward them and pain over the freedoms that they themselves had missed out on. They speculated that they were unable to bear such feelings and had consequently become depressed.

We brainstormed together, eventually wondering if women in their grandmothers' generation might unconsciously expect contempt from young women with such different values and expectations. Per-haps it would help a depressed grandmother if her granddaughter could express her admiration for how well she had coped with such confin-ing cultural demands and indicate her appreciation of the sacrifices required by such an adaptation. They agreed that this had some prom-ise. My main reflection about this conversation was that I would never get such a question from an American audience of therapists, many of whom would be sorry that grandma was depressed but feel no per-sonal responsibility to relieve her pain. In addition, I suspect that many Americans, upon hearing about these therapists' concern for someone in their extended family, would insensitively conclude that the clini-cians who asked the question had failed to separate enough from their families of origin.

In the United States, professionals have frequently misunderstood patients from collectivist cultures as pathologically dependent or prob-lematically unseparated from their families of origin (Gherovici & Christian, 2018; Tummala-Narra, 2016). In complementary fashion, therapists in more collectivist societies sometimes pathologize Western patients, seeing them as selfish or self-centered. Such a narrow vision can apply also to subgroups that deviate from the dominant cultural tone (Sue, 2010). Because of their more extensive experience with both therapeutic work and life in general, supervisors may see clinical populations through a wider societal lens, a lens that their mentees will need.

VITALITY

D. W. Winnicott is said to have quipped, "A person can be normal without being alive." Psychoanalytic therapists hope to help patients find their curiosity, enthusiasm, and passion (see Panizza, 2014). For a long time, we have tried to conceptualize individuals who lack vitality, who seem to be going through the motions of life without fully living it. In trying to capture the psychology of such people, Helene Deutsch (1942) suggested the concept of the "as-if personality," Winnicott (1960) described the "false self," Joyce McDougall (1980) coined the term "normopath," and Christopher Bollas (1987) depicted "normotic" psychologies. Relational analysts might construe clients who are describable in such terms as in a prolonged state of dissociation from their affective life (e.g., Stern, 2009). Lacanians might note their lack of "jouissance." At the extreme end of the continuum of internal deadness is André Green's (1993) "dead mother syndrome" (Kohon, 1999; Mucci, 2018), in which it is posited that there is no internalization of early maternal excitement about one's existence.

The as-if-ness of such individuals may strike us as similar to a state of anhedonic depression, but they experience it as a chronic fact of life rather than as a deviation from a state in which their existence had meaning, purpose, and emotional richness. It includes alexithymia and the state of mind that has more recently been identified as "affective agnosia" (Lane, Weihs, Herring, Hishaw, & Smith, 2015). Perhaps recent global trends (mass culture, dizzyingly swift change, instant communication, bureaucracy, mobility, consumerism, etc.) can be blamed for the fact that many of us lack an inner source of enlivenment and feel as if we are acting in someone else's play, like the main character in *The Truman Show*.

In contemporary life it is easy to feel the pressures of external forces at the expense of internal ones. Substances may play a central role, too, in a lack of vitality. Not only do people who feel dead inside seek substances like cocaine and amphetamines that will energize them, but they also learn eventually, even after becoming reliably sober, that internal deadness is a common aftermath of addiction, which highjacks the dopamine system. Boredom can thus be a major risk factor for substance use disorders and addiction and may also be a torment of early sobriety (Washton & Zweben, 2006).

Rarely do incoming patients complain explicitly about an absence of vitality: A person who has never felt inner aliveness has no way to know that something is missing. In the parallel process, supervisees may have trouble describing "what is wrong" with clients who lack vitality. Such patients tend to complain of other, more concrete issues, such as an eating disorder or addiction (about which the therapist typically has a hard time engaging them). Often, they are sent by others. A man came to me saying his wife thought he needed treatment because he never expressed interest or enthusiasm. I failed to engage him adequately and, when he quit after a few sessions, blamed myself for not being a good-enough therapist. An empathic supervisor could have helped me at that point, either to keep the patient or to lighten up on myself or both.

Supervisors are more likely than less experienced clinicians to pick up the fact that "there's nobody home" or "this person sleepwalks through life." Newer clinicians may be relieved that the odd disconnectedness they were feeling is not due to their own deficit in empathy or skill; it is related to the patient's absence of inner animation. Whatever the presenting problem, once this lifelessness has been named, it can become a clinical focus. The therapist can be helped to assist the patient in finding sincere emotions, interests, and motives. Usually, at some point in any person's life, there was *some* passion—even if it was for baseball stats or video games or celebrity sightings—that the clinician and client can jointly try to recapture and from which a sense of vitality may slowly expand.

ACCEPTANCE, FORGIVENESS, AND GRATITUDE

Psychotherapy is not simply about changing one's behavior; it is also about accepting what cannot be changed. Coming to terms with an irreversible loss requires a grief process, sometimes a long one. Mourning seems to be nature's way of helping us adapt to life's most painful wounds. Our loss may be of a person, a possession, a beloved animal, or a place and way of being, such as one's homeland and the culture and language that were part of it. Or it may be the permanent passing of one's youth, one's prior state of health, one's job, or one's previous expectations or illusions. It may involve grieving the downside of a decision that had mostly positive effects, such as a choice to divorce or change gender.

In the literature influenced by the positive psychology movement and related current social trends, there is been a resurgence of attention to the value of acceptance, gratitude, and forgiveness, attitudes that religious groups have always emphasized but that secular cultures often have not. Perhaps one contributing factor to contemporary interests in Buddhism and mindfulness may be a widespread need for their focus on what simply *is* rather than on the constant striving for *what might be* that Western consumerist ideologies promote. Such wisdom is critical to psychotherapy, whose core values are sometimes at odds with the assumptions of its surrounding commercial culture. In the psychoanalytic literature, there has been an increased interest in wisdom generally, and in topics like forgiveness (e.g., Mucci, 2013; Siassi, 2013).

Clinicians need to learn from their supervisors how to foster serenity and forbearance in the face of life's difficulties. Simply reducing overt symptoms may leave this area untouched. A man who feels less anxious but who is still holding a deep grudge is only marginally better off than when he came to treatment; a woman who feels entitled to all her advantages rather than feeling grateful for them will have a recurrently resentful life whenever she confronts limitations. Supervisors have a critical role in helping clinicians to bear their patient's suffering when it involves experiences that cannot be undone. Although it never fully goes away, grief does eventually soften, and the mourning process enriches those who can tolerate going through it. Therapists who offer reassurances, reframing, behavioral goals, and other distractions are not likely to do the important work of bearing witness to a process of deep healing.

Sitting with suffering tends to make new clinicians worry that they are not "doing enough." They need help with their omnipotent wishes to be able to "cure" rather than help people endure life's inevitable hardships. They need supervisors who can model a comfort with making mistakes (acceptance of one's limitations), can respond to the therapist's mistakes without condemnation (forgiveness), and can attest to the realistic pleasures that come with being a therapist (gratitude). Psychoanalytic supervision involves clarity about what can be changed versus what must simply be accepted and grieved. The hopes of newer therapists to be able to do the impossible need to be challenged; otherwise, clinicians can never fully appreciate what *is* possible in therapy and how precious such movement can be to their clients.

LOVE, WORK, AND PLAY

Erik Erikson (1950) reported that when Freud was asked his perspective on the overall goal of psychoanalytic treatment, he responded that therapy should create or restore the capacity "to love and to work." The late Bertram Karon once told me that Richard Sterba claimed to have heard Freud say something similar, but in this recollection, he had added "and also enjoyment, of course." I am translating this mental health ideal into "love, work, and play." It could be argued that most of the capacities I have listed above can be subsumed under these topics, or—more reasonably, I think—that the ability to love, work, and play depends on them.

By love, psychoanalysts do not necessarily mean conventional notions of heterosexual marriage and parenthood. The capacity to love that we try to support and expand in therapy has two central elements: (1) deeply caring about the people in one's life *as they really are* (rather than as one wishes they were, i.e., the difference between mature love and idealization) and (2) the capacity for devotion. By work, we do not necessarily mean holding a job, but doing something useful that has personal meaning, including unpaid nurturing, a religious or political vocation, or volunteer work. The meaning of one's work can be anything from providing for one's family, even via a job one hates, to the intrinsic satisfactions of artists, scholars, and others who love their work for its own sake. By play, we mean the childhood capacities for imaginative expression, humor, and normal rough-and-tumble interaction (Panksepp & Biven, 2012) as well as adult involvements such as sexual activity, sports, hobbies, games, music, theater, dance, and the arts.

CONCLUDING COMMENTS

These 10 areas amount to psychological vital signs that psychodynamic clinicians teach their supervisors to monitor. Because they involve cognitive and emotional achievements that a difficult history may have prevented, many patients do not depict their problems in these terms. We cannot imagine what we have never had. If I have never been able to trust (attachment security), or soothe myself when stressed (affect regulation), or appreciate someone else's state of mind (mentalization), I cannot conceive of doing so. If I have never had reason to trust, I may see a clinician as naive for thinking trust is reasonable; if I take personally my partner's idiosyncrasies, I may pressure my therapist to change the partner; if I have not become friendly with solitude, I may be unable to imagine that state as anything other than terrifying. Often, supervisors need to help therapists find ways to help clients begin to envisage such capacities in the first place.

In this chapter I have reviewed areas of clinical growth and healing that go beyond symptom reduction and that are basic to overall psychological wellness. I have organized this territory under the rubrics of attachment security; feelings of continuity; a sense of agency; realistic and reliable self-esteem; affect tolerance and regulation; reflective function and mentalization; comfort with both self-direction and communality; vitality; acceptance of what cannot be changed; and increased capacity for love, work, and play. Most psychoanalytic mentors keep these vital signs in mind in whatever language they have learned to think about them, and they convey to supervisees their knowledge of particular domains as they apply to particular patients. I am hoping that by having listed them and elaborated briefly on these different mental functions, I have been helpful to supervisors in noticing areas that they may need to address with clinicians who are trying to learn to think and work psychoanalytically.

Chapter Four

■　■　■　■

Individual Supervision
and Consultation

Most psychodynamic clinicians would likely say that their early supervision was more critical to their development than their course work and readings. Guest and Beutler (1988) found long ago that initial experiences in supervision remain alive in therapists' minds and are influential for years and even decades afterward. In the supervisory relationship we learn to formulate each patient's dynamics, conceptualize what is going on in the clinical moment, increase our skills at listening and intervening, engage in reverie and notice our internal associations, assimilate professional knowledge, monitor our strengths and vulnerabilities, learn about our blind spots, and adapt our personalities to the art of therapy. Supervisors naturally vary in their skills in addressing these different areas, and the wise supervisee learns to take from each mentor what is most valuable in that person's repertoire.

A premise of this chapter is that most clinicians have a natural human curiosity and a deep wish to keep learning and improving their effectiveness. Most supervisees thus thrive on opportunities to increase their knowledge and develop their clinical skills. This assumption parallels the core psychoanalytic conviction that patients, however conflicted they may be about changing, have an internal drive toward psychological health that makes the difficult work of therapy possible. Psychodynamic consultation attempts to help clinicians enjoy and value a process that supervisors hope they will want to engage in throughout their professional lives. It is a cardinal analytic belief that the job of a mentor, whether a therapist, consultant, or supervisor, is to remove obstacles from learning and provide psychological nutrition for normal maturational processes.

Although research on therapists' evaluation of their supervision is still relatively sparse (Eubanks et al., 2019; Feinstein, Huhn, & Yager, 2015; O'Donovan & Kavanagh, 2014), a substantial empirical literature is beginning to emerge on the topic that complements existing writing that has been more qualitative and personal (e.g., Rock, 1997). Two recent, coordinated issues of *Training and Education in Professional Psychology* (Callahan & Love, 2019) and the *Journal of Psychotherapy Integration* (Callahan, 2020) have been devoted to accounts of supervisees' experiences of their training. Finally, the voices of the recipients of supervision are joining those of the people entrusted with their clinical education.

I have heard about experiences of supervision that run the gamut from extremely helpful to outright damaging (see Dr. Lamia's brief account in Chapter 1). Empirical studies also attest to this range (e.g., Bambling, 2000; Ellis, 2017; Ellis et al., 2014; Gray, Ladany, Walker, & Ancis, 2001; Henry, Schahct, Strupp, Butler, & Binder, 1993). It is my impression that most psychodynamic therapists recall their formative supervision as a kind of holding environment (Winnicott, 1953) in which they felt respected, supported, and filled with a rich stew of information, theories, problem-solving strategies, expansion of their empathy, new perspectives on their countertransferences, and other nourishing ingredients. At the other end of the spectrum, some remember supervision as torture and are only too glad at the current time to be either unsupervised or working with a handpicked consultant who will not replicate the torments of their training. In this chapter I focus on some elements of effective individual supervision, hoping to increase the instances in which supervision is assimilated more as the former rather than the latter experience.

ESTABLISHING AND MAINTAINING THE SUPERVISORY ALLIANCE

A strong alliance is foundational to effective supervision and also to the identity development of the supervisee as a clinician. Increasingly, the empirical literature, both quantitative (e.g., Geller, Farber, & Schaffer, 2010; Nagell et al., 2014; Watkins, 2011) and qualitative (e.g., Cucco, 2020; Mammen, 2020), supports that long-standing psychoanalytic lore. The best way I know to create a strong supervisory alliance is to be useful to supervisees, and in the process to be respectful of their emotional intelligence, potential intuitive skill, and good intentions. The following sections discuss some elements involved in the mutual construction of a strong alliance, with an emphasis on the supervisor's role in making this possible.

The Supervisory Contract

In the beginning of any course of supervision or consultation, both parties should clarify what they will be doing together. Different supervisors have different preferences for the presentation of clinical material (e.g., watching videos, reading process notes, or inviting the student's report of what happened). They also have different preferences for whether to follow one patient in depth or to consult on multiple cases as the student feels the need. The training program for which they supervise may also have rules about such issues (e.g., most analytic institutes want advanced candidates to present single cases in depth, one per supervisor; graduate programs generally require that every patient the student sees be talked about regularly with a supervisor even if the work seems to be going well).

One interesting newer approach to supervision is Feinstein's cognitive apprenticeship model (Feinstein, 2020; Feinstein et al., 2015; Feinstein & Yager, 2013). This empirically tested method involves the supervisee's observation of a supervisor's therapy session with a patient, followed by a discussion of the supervisor's orienting conceptualizations and rationales for interventions. Then the trainee works similarly with a patient while receiving supervisory feedback (via Bluetooth connection or the supervisor's presence in the room), both during and after the session. Live supervision is familiar to family therapists but mostly alien to psychoanalysts, who worry about splitting the patient's transference. Despite such concerns, and despite early resistance from supervisors of all orientations, Feinstein and his coauthors found that once their reluctant colleagues tried it, they found live supervision in an apprenticeship format to be effective and gratifying. Patients were mostly cooperative and appreciative of the extra attention, and trainees, although initially apprehensive, reported benefiting from the approach. I am not personally familiar with this way of working, but I am impressed with Feinstein's results.

In the mental health field, we have made significant advances in the area of consent for treatment, but not so much with respect to the contract for supervision. In most treatment consent forms, the patient signs on to the therapist's arrangements about scheduling, payment, and cancellation policies, as well as to summaries about patient rights, confidentiality and its legal exceptions, and so on. In supervision and consultation, contractual consent is usually verbal rather than written, but some parallel considerations apply. In the first meeting, supervisors need to specify what they will expect, how they like to work, and, if relevant, how they will approach any reporting about their evaluation of the clinician to third parties. The supervisee should make clear what he or she hopes to gain from the experience and should have ample opportunity to ask questions and share concerns. Because supervisees are prone to idealization of their clinical mentors, especially early in their careers, and will need to replace the pedestal eventually with internalizations of realistic professional competence, it can be helpful when supervisors comment to them self-reflectively on their own individual strengths and limitations.

The supervisory contract should be revisable over time, as the supervisee's interests or status changes and also in response to the pair's developing an understanding of what kinds of help a particular therapist needs. In their early meetings, the two parties need to clarify the expectations of each one. Just as, in therapy, it is vital to understand the problem for which the patient came and the kind of help being sought, in supervision, it is important to be on the same page about the general focus and direction of the work. By the time both people have accepted the specifics of their arrangement, the supervisee should be confident that there will be no surprises down the road about supervisory practices and reciprocal responsibilities.

Especially when supervision sessions will not be directly observed, the contract should specify what information the supervisor expects when the less experienced colleague presents a case. Here is my own list of questions for supervisees to address, which can usually be communicated verbally rather than in writing:

- "What is the clinical problem or issue with which you want help?"

- "Who is the patient (age, relationship status, gender and sexual identifications, ethnic/racial/class/religious identifications, current situation, physical presentation, general attitude toward the therapist)?"

- "How long and at what frequency have you seen the patient? How did he or she come to you? What is the person's prior experience with therapy, if any?"

- "What is the problem for which the patient came for help?"

- "When did that problem start, and how does the patient understand why it started then?"

- "What is the short version of the patient's childhood history? How does he or she describe caregivers, siblings, and other important influences? How reliable and comprehensive does the patient's account seem to you?"

- "What is the emotional tone of the therapy?"

- "How do you find yourself feeling with the patient?"

Formulating Realistic Therapy Goals for Patients

There is empirical support (e.g., Lehrman-Waterman & Ladany, 2001) for long-standing clinical observations that goal setting promotes a solid supervisory alliance and supervisee satisfaction. Goals for psychodynamic treatments involve both symptom relief and improvement in the areas I have summarized in the previous chapter. Mental health is not unidimensional; for example, high affect tolerance or vitality can coexist with low self-esteem or lack of agency. Patients differ on which vital signs need to be monitored. Whenever possible (though when developmental achievements that the therapist and supervisor are capable of envisaging involve capacities the patient cannot yet imagine, it may not be possible), the client should participate in formulating treatment goals that go beyond symptom reduction. One of the first tasks of the supervisee with any patient will therefore be to articulate treatment goals to which the patient can sign on. Thus, supervisors and supervisees need to share a vision of what would constitute significant progress for each client. This can be trickier than it appears.

For example, there may be implicit or explicit differences between supervisor and supervisee about how serious any patient's problem is. In my experience, unless a person's self-presentation clearly accords with the DSM or ICD diagnostic criteria for borderline personality disorder or a psychotic disorder, beginning therapists often fail to recognize severe psychological disturbance. Graduate programs tend to warn students not to overpathologize, but they rarely alert them to the dangers of underpathologizing. Especially if a person is bright, privileged, and competent in many areas, students tend not to pick up right away on how primitive their defenses are, how deeply distrustful they may be, or how internally empty their subjective world is. They tend to identify with areas in which the client is like them (e.g., smart, socially adept, holding similar values or interests) and unconsciously infer that their level of psychological wellness is also similar. It can be shocking to beginning therapists to realize how many seriously troubled people inhabit the world and how deep is the suffering of those they have signed up to help. One of my younger supervisees once remarked, "Growing up, if I had known how messed up so many people are, I would have spent my childhood being either terrified of what's out there or guilty about my family's sanity."

On the other hand, some supervisees are surprised, and often chagrined, to discover that qualities they have considered "normal" are widely regarded by therapists as pathological. Examples might include assumptions that all married couples fight angrily, that no one likes being alone, that all parents criticize their children unendingly, that everyone is obsessed with physical perfection, that an adolescence without binge drinking is unheard of, and so on. We all generalize about normality from our family of origin and our peer group, and in the Internet age, we can find whole communities of people who share our assumptions and cannot imagine any state of affairs that differs from the one in which they grew up. Such experiences in cyber silos tend to reinforce older learning.

It is painful for supervisees when qualities in themselves that they believed were universal are framed as problematic. Their awareness of such discrepancies between what they have taken for granted and what clinicians generally regard as normal or healthy often arises from their supervisory experience, not so much from intentionally didactic commentary as from matter-of-fact remarks or questions (e.g., "Why do you think your client falls into helpless tears rather than negotiating for what she wants?" or "How do you understand this man's conviction that apologizing is not 'masculine'?" or "What has made your client think that being smarter than other people is the ticket to satisfaction in life?"). After noticing their own normalization of problematic phenomena, they have to face anxieties about whether they are healthy enough to be a therapist. In my experience, they usually are, but they nonetheless have to cope with shame about previously unacknowledged limitations.

Returning to the general topic of novice clinicians' tendencies to see patients as healthier than they are, I have found that students' prior training in empathic listening and the temperamental and psychological qualities that originally disposed them toward becoming therapists incline them to seek similarity and shrink from seeing others as different in a negative direction. Their tendency to see a patient's strengths, at the expense of noticing some troubling weaknesses, has many benefits, including the expectation that they can help, which contributes to patients' hopes for relief from psychological pain. And yet, if students lack a realistic idea of a client's level of psychological organization, they run the risk of pursuing goals that are unattainable in either the near or distant future. Patients can be deeply dismayed by their failure to achieve such goals, and therapists can draw the conclusion that there is something wrong with them as clinicians for not succeeding as they have imagined.

This problem is one of the unintended consequences of the current emphasis on evidence-based treatments. Such therapies are valuable, but they are often empirically tested and validated with the highest-functioning patients in any given symptomatic category. In studies of comparative treatments, researchers generally weed out participants with "comorbidities," who tend to be precisely the more "difficult" or "treatment-resistant" patients that therapists need the most guidance to treat. As a practical matter, mentally healthier individuals are also more cooperative with researchers' agendas and less likely to drop out of a study or miss appointments, and so they are overrepresented in the data that are analyzed in randomized controlled trials.

On the basis of such outcome research, beginning therapists' professors may have definitively told them, among other things, that exposure is a proven treatment for obsessive–compulsive disorders. They are right about that. But they may have gone further to insist that it is the "best practice" or the "treatment of choice" or even that it is unethical to work in any other way with individuals who have obsessions and compulsions. In recent years, I have heard many accounts of such opinions asserted by people whose clinical experience has been minimal. Their confident convictions can leave students helpless when they meet patients with long-standing obsessive–compulsive disorder and many comorbidities, whose personality organization may be at the borderline or psychotic level of severity (Kernberg, 1984).

Both professional lore and common sense suggest that exposure works much better with patients who can understand that their ruminations and rituals are crazy, who can recall a time before they had them, whose family members did not model and reinforce them, and who can appreciate both consciously and unconsciously that the therapist is well intentioned. After graduating from academic programs, therapists must work with many people who would have been excluded from clinical trials, who privately believe they may be in grave danger without their obsessions and compulsions, who cannot remember when they did not have them, whose caregivers had similar preoccupations, and who fear that a clinician might somehow harm them. Such patients tend to respond to exposure with terror and/or profound resistance. Urging them too soon or too uncritically into exposure paradigms is a setup for the patient's disillusionment about the value of treatment and the therapist's feelings of failure and burnout. This is only one example among many of the consequences of the current disconnect between what can be easily researched and what is clinically relevant.

It is not always easy for a supervisor to convey to newer therapists that they may be misjudging a patient's level of psychological dysfunction. Seasoned mentors frequently encounter resistance to their efforts, however gentle, to point out the depth of a client's difficulties. Often, they are misperceived as regarding treatment as hopeless or as being critical or dismissive of the patient (admittedly, this can sometimes be an accurate perception, but I am talking here about instances when it is not). To the extent that newer therapists identify with any patient, they can feel uncomfortably exposed and apprehensive in the face of the supervisor's focus on the person's more primitive dynamics.

We all have archaic mental processes, but the point needs to be made to supervisees that many patients lack access to more mature adaptations; it is the absence of these adaptations rather than the presence of more primitive operations that suggests more severe psychopathology. It is a delicate balance to try, on one hand, to increase supervisees' capacity to see in themselves the kinds of issues they see in patients (a process that can increase their empathy and respect) and, on the other hand, to note the ways in which such similarities do not indicate that the patient's and therapist's respective difficulties in maintaining their sanity are equivalent. It is important to help clinicians appreciate the universal tendencies that they share with even the craziest patient and at the same time not minimize the patient's level of damage.

I remember a beginning student who was by temperament a gifted empath. She was truly puzzled when I suggested that the man she had begun to treat for an anxiety disorder had some psychotic features, including ideas of reference and terrifying annihilation anxiety. She became uncomfortable when I observed that his political ideas had a paranoid feel and were predicated on the defense of splitting, with no capacity to reflect on his splits. Her political views were similar to his (and so were mine), but she differed radically from her patient in that she was able to understand that her political enemies were not monsters but included individuals who might be well intentioned. She was able, largely because of her mature capacity to tell the truth even to an authority in an evaluative role, to disclose her worries that I was critical of her politics and insensitive to the issues about which she and her patient cared deeply.

Because of these worries, she had begun to feel a bit unsafe with me, a reaction we were able to see as paralleling her client's deep sense of distrust. Like her, he was very bright; she found it counterintuitive that such intellectual firepower could coexist with emotional fragility and psychotic anxiety. And given her empathic tilt, she experienced his primitive idealization of her as comparable to the reality-based trust she had often felt toward admired others, whereas his idealization had been immediate and based on a primitive merger fantasy that she was in every way a soul mate. He had a history of idealizing and then traumatically devaluing those he had depended on. The therapist eventually realized that making an attachment with this man that was solid enough to keep him out of the hospital was a therapeutic "win," even if he still suffered some anxiety. Her tendency to identify with him was a positive factor in his treatment, in that he thrived in the atmosphere of her egalitarian attitude. But in supervision, she and I had to process the fact that what she and he had in common did not extend to their sharing the same level of overall wellness.

A male supervisee I once worked with was assigned a female patient with "anger management issues" and a history of antisocial behavior. This included having deliberately (and without remorse) tormented her much younger siblings, having reacted with sadistic glee when one of her adolescent rivals was raped, and having sold drugs to friends who were now addicted ("That's their problem"). She behaved in a charming, seductive way with my supervisee—never enough to be accused of "inappropriate" behavior, but enough to make him feel that, despite his knowledge of her checkered background, if she and he were not in the roles of therapist and patient, they could be close friends or lovers. Like the clinician in the previous example, even though his moral faculties were quite intact, my student found himself feeling deeply identified with, and attracted to, this evidently calculating woman.

This man was greatly helped by a combination of group and individual supervision. When he began talking in the group about the beauty, sensitivity, and intelligence of his client, presenting her as regrettably misunderstood by everyone else, his peers began to be visibly uncomfortable. One participant challenged him in a "man-to-man" blunt way, teasing him about how skillfully his patient had fed his narcissism. When he became defensive, the other group members chimed in more tactfully, sharing their curiosity about the fact that although he presented his patient as lovely, they found themselves not liking her. He was not entirely talked out of his overall formulation (she was misunderstood and he was her lone and righteous champion), but soon his client asked him to lie to the clinic to get her a lower fee, and he began to admit the possibility of an antisocial tinge to her charm.

As further interactions confirmed the group's intuitions, he talked in individual supervision about his feelings of humiliation for having been so gullible. I responded with stories about instances in my own work history when psychopathic individuals have "gotten over" on me. I characterized his vulnerability to her manipulation as the downside of his openness to her experience, a compassionate position and mindset that would generally serve him well as a therapist but that psychopathic patients can be geniuses at exploiting. He and I came to the conclusion that he was projecting his own integrity onto the patient, denying her antisocial traits because they were so disturbing to imagine.

I noted that we are all mammals, with a potential for predatory ruth-lessness, and suggested that if he could find that potential in himself, he might be able see it more easily elsewhere. In dissociating from his own capacity for psychopathy, he might be blinding himself to Machiavellian tendencies in anyone he cared about. Another possible risk of denying one's own antisocial potential is that when psychopathic features can-not be ignored in another person, we tend to see him or her entirely as "other," as monstrous deviations from humanity. We also talked about paying attention to countertransference reactions, which can include being besotted by a client as well as feeling "played," "pinned against the ropes," or chilled and "under the thumb" of a manipulator (Evans, 2011; Meloy, 1988; Mulay, Kelly, & Cain, 2017). Then we talked about the general principles of how to exert therapeutic influence on someone whose psychology was organized around power rather than around love and attachment (McWilliams, 2011).

A converse problem to the tendency of newer supervisees to under-pathologize clients is to overpathologize themselves. This response is a psychological parallel to the "medical student syndrome," in which the smallest bodily glitch alarms an aspiring doctor about the possibility of a fatal illness. Avoiding either–or thinking is particularly important when making inferences about a client's level of functioning and con-sequent realistic treatment goals. Supervisors need to convey that all patients have weaknesses *and* strengths; they can be very psychologi-cally disturbed *and* remarkably resilient; clinicians' dynamics that par-allel those of their patients can be both interferences *and* assets to the therapy process.

A mutual assessment of level of severity (Kernberg, 1984; Lingiardi & McWilliams, 2017) has critical implications not only for the choice of treatment approach and specification of ultimate goals, but also for what kinds of developments can be noted as evidence of progress (or lack thereof) in an ongoing therapy. Without such an assessment, it is easy to get that inference wrong. One of my supervisees, for example, tended to project his own level of agency onto a female patient who was having difficulty leaving a troubled relationship. His assumption that this should not be hard to do got in the way of his appreciating the import of an instance when his client had, for the first time, told her boyfriend that it hurt her feelings when he criticized her. This was a major move toward self-advocacy on her part, but because of my supervisee's implicit belief that she was capable of his own level of autonomy, he framed it dismissively as a "baby step." His missing the significance of her achievement deprived her of the experience of being witnessed having done something very hard, and it deprived him of realistic evidence of his competence. Another supervisee was appalled when her 7-year-old client yelled "Fuck you!" at her even though this outburst amounted to substantial progress in a child who had been selectively mute for months.

Supervisees need to learn that the rate of treatment progress is hard to predict, no matter how extensive the original assessment. Both anecdotally and empirically (e.g., Seligman, 1995), treatment frequency and length have been associated with therapy effectiveness. We can thus tell trainees with some confidence that what can be expected in short-term or spaced-out treatment will be less than what can be accomplished in longer and more intensive therapies. But beyond that, reasonable expectations for many psychological changes depend on a range of factors, many of which cannot be assessed at the beginning of a treatment, such as the patient's level of motivation once the work starts; or how good the fit will feel to both parties; or whether friends, family members, and the fates will reinforce or undermine positive changes in the client.

In the mid-20th century, much attention was devoted to trying to assess at the outset of treatment whether a given person was "analyzable." Despite earnest efforts, no one ever came up with a foolproof formula for evaluating analyzability (Erle, 1979; Frosch, 2006; Karon, 2002; Peebles-Kleiger, Horwitz, Kleiger, & Waugaman, 2006). Clinical lore abounds about "beginner's zeal," or how newcomers to the field have succeeded with patients that the experienced staff members at their place of work had regarded as untreatable. Supervision requires a subtle balance between supporting the therapeutic ambitions of younger clinicians and at the same time tempering their pursuit of the impossible, so that they can reasonably appraise their progress with each client.

I want to end this section by commenting on the difference between treatment goals and life goals. Ernst Ticho (1972) originally wrote about this distinction in ways I found helpful as a novice clinician. Treatment goals include areas that are influenceable by work on the self; life goals depend heavily on factors outside one's control. Therapy goals thus might include reducing perfectionism, increasing realistic self-esteem, resolving an internal conflict, making a difficult choice, mourning a painful loss, and so on. Life goals include, for example, finding a partner or spouse, getting a good job, or becoming a parent. They may be attained more easily when therapy goals have met, but they are not themselves treatment goals. Clinicians cannot promise that at the end of the therapy there will be a partner, a job, or a baby; for those aspirations, too much depends on external circumstances. Newer therapists need supervisory help in not signing on to pursue a client's life goals, but instead in reconceptualizing and reframing the clinical task as internally directed work that may increase the probability of achieving such goals.

Promoting Openness and Honesty

After agreeing on the ground rules, therapist and supervisor need to work on creating an atmosphere in which the supervisee can be as forthcoming as possible about his or her work. If the sessions have been videotaped and watched together (or audiotaped and listened to together), the issue of the supervisor's knowing what "really" went on in a session is less problematic for him or her and, simply via exposure, potentially more conducive to the supervisee's eventual comfort in being witnessed. But it also involves more anxiety for the trainee that supervisors need to appreciate. The question of how the supervisee feels about being scrutinized is always worth exploring.

For psychoanalytically oriented practitioners, a core effort underlying both psychotherapy and supervision is the creation of an interpersonal space that allows as much honesty as human beings are capable of with each other (cf. Thompson, 2004). This is a lot easier when a clinician seeks mentorship voluntarily, when the supervisee can choose the consultant, and when there is not an evaluating authority to whom that consultant reports. I address some nuances of the supervisor's responsibility to training programs and the public in Chapters 6 and 7, but I mention the topic here because such situations complicate the possibilities for honesty for both supervisee and supervisor. Often, such issues cannot be transcended because to the supervisee so much hinges on being positively evaluated. Showing one's limitations feels dangerous. But at least this reality can be named and understood explicitly, and I think it is critical to model frankness by naming that elephant in the consulting room.

Even when supervision is free of the complications of oversight and involuntariness, there are internal and relational dynamics on both sides that complicate efforts to be candid. Supervisees want to learn but also want to be seen as competent therapists, and they may have practical worries about whether the supervisor will refer patients to them or recommend them to colleagues looking to refer clients. They want to improve their knowledge while not appearing too ignorant of what they should already know. For supervisors, the complications arise mostly from concerns not to hurt the supervisee's feelings.

Whatever the challenges to a forthright supervisory relationship may be, here are some ways I have learned to help therapists become more comfortable opening up to me. First, I disclose a lot about my own slow path to learning, emphasizing my misunderstandings and mistakes and what has helped me to improve in whatever area I am seeing a problem in the supervisee. Second, I try to remember to ask frequently if there are any matters the supervisee finds hard to talk about or notices he or she is avoiding. Third, I frequently ask for feedback about how the supervision is going from the perspective of the supervisee.

If the supervisee seems ingratiating or avoidant, I may try to "drill down," as cognitive-behavioral therapists say, on specific areas. For example, have I said anything with which the supervisee has disagreed but did not feel able to tell me? Am I being sensitive enough to issues of culture, race, sexuality, religion, and similar factors in the clinical work? Researchers (e.g., Cabaniss et al., 2001; Ladany, Hill, Corbett, & Nutt, 1996; Mehr, Ladany, & Caskie, 2015; Strømme & Gullestad, 2012; Yourman & Farber, 1996) have consistently found that supervisees withhold important information from supervisors. One thing I am careful *not* to do is to pursue information about the supervisee's background or psychology that is legitimately private and might feel too exposing; for example, I would not ask whether the mentee has ever struggled with an addiction or has a history of sexual abuse. But I do try, as I discuss in the next chapter, to make supervisees feel safe enough to offer information of that sort voluntarily. Doing so can increase self-acceptance, openness to learning, and integration of their emotional experiences with their intellectual understandings.

Finally, as part of the effort to encourage supervisees to consider that they are in a relationship in which they are free to disagree, I ask them explicitly for criticism of my work as a supervisor. Parenthetically, I am not fond of evaluation forms as an ongoing way of assessing the evolution of the supervisory relationship; these surveys deflect from frank, face-to-face conversations and permit the supervisee's negative feelings to be displaced onto a questionnaire. Such forms have an important place in research and in programs that need to evaluate supervisors systematically, but they are not a substitute for a direct conversation about the supervisor's limitations as the supervisee experiences them. Exemplifying the willingness to be vulnerable and a preference for candor over comfort are key supervisory attitudes for mentees to internalize and generalize to their clinical practice.

Supervisees may have come to their professional calling from backgrounds in which they were the parentified child in their family of origin, and see themselves as having taken on the sensitive family-therapist role originally depicted by Alice Miller (1975) that resonated with so many practitioners and made her book on the "drama of the gifted child" an instant hit in its time. Their automatic default may thus be to try to take care of the supervisor's narcissistic needs at the cost of their own forthrightness. This would be a good dynamic for them to know about and work on. It is hard for people who were raised to support parental self-esteem to question authority. Just as therapists need to learn to ask patients about negative feelings toward themselves, mentors should be able not only to tolerate criticism, but also to invite it.

Supervisors should give supervisees an unambiguous message to the effect that because they are the ones in the room with the patient, they may know more than the supervisor about the possible consequences of alternative ways of dealing with a clinical problem. In a difference of opinion between supervisor and supervisee, unless there is a clear ethical problem with what the treating therapist feels is the right thing to do, I believe that supervisees should be encouraged to try out their own ideas about what is clinically best in any situation. I take this position partly because I think they will not be able to do anything else with authenticity, partly because they are the ones in the physical presence of the patient, receiving all the person's nonverbal communications, and partly because I never really learned anything myself without first trying out what made sense to me and making my own mistakes. But more important, by implementing what seems to them the proper intervention, mentees will either learn from an error or prove the supervisor wrong, either of which will contribute to their growth.

Once when I was leading a discussion for a group of psychologists who provide unremunerated supervision to the students in our program at Rutgers, I asked them why they were willing to contribute their time *pro bono.* In addition to their many comments about enjoying our students, they agreed that they learned, even from these novice clinicians, many new ways of relating therapeutically to patients. Without having created an environment in which their students felt free to disagree with them, all those opportunities for the supervisor's own professional enrichment would have been foreclosed. Therapists tend to like having multiple ideas about how to approach any resistant pattern of emotion, cognition, or behavior, because they can easily feel that their usual methods are getting stale and are losing their power to influence their clients. Exposure to the solutions of other therapists, no matter how inexperienced, expands one's clinical repertoire.

ADDRESSING RESISTANCES TO LEARNING

Even though supervision is not therapy, there may be times, especially early in the process, when the supervisor has to address transferences and defenses that get in the way of optimal learning. Some of these resistances are almost universal in supervision. For example, there are some defenses that issue from the depressive dynamics (Hyde, 2009) that I mentioned in Chapter 1. Many clinicians are hard on themselves internally, and they project their self-criticism (their harsh superegos) onto mentors. Expectations of disapproval, an inability to distinguish helpful suggestions from accusations of ineptitude, and shame about ignorance and presumed errors are common.

In the next chapter I discuss ways to make a group supervision setting feel safe enough for participants to be open about their work. Most of those ideas apply equally to individual supervision. But in one-on-one situations, because a supervisee cannot so easily hide or feel support from peers if the supervisor is critical, he or she may feel an even more excruciating sense of exposure and anxiety about disapproval than would pertain in a group. In Chapter 1, I noted that a common defense against fears of being sadistically exposed by a supervisor is the masochistic strategy of attacking oneself preemptively. Thus, many supervisees begin virtually every meeting by confessing one putative error after another, making the implicit plea, "Please don't attack me! I'm already attacking myself, so the job is already done." The supervisee is making the tacit calculation that a mentor who is poised to condemn will back off. If criticism turns out *not* to be the supervisor's intent, the student reasons, nothing has been lost by the strategy of self-attack.

But defensive self-criticism does waste time and energy that could be devoted to learning, and it can be irritating to the mentor, who wants to support the supervisee and instead feels defensively distanced and misunderstood as a potential bully. My preferred way of dealing with this pattern, as I noted previously, is to name the masochistic defense when I think I am seeing it, to say that I "get it" because I also behaved that way with my early supervisors, and to urge the mentee to take the risk of simply saying what happened without encasing the clinical data in an armor of self-criticism and penitence.

A common defense in early supervisions that do not rely on video or audio records is speaking rather vaguely about general concepts rather than stating what one explicitly said and did. For example, "I expressed support," or "I mirrored the patient's feelings." Just as with clients who speak vaguely (e.g., answering "weird," or "tense" when the therapist inquires how they feel about something), with supervisees who hide behind abstractions and generalizations, the supervisor may have to keep reiterating, albeit kindly, queries such as "What did you actually say?" or "What is your idea of giving support?" or "Which of the patient's conflicting feelings did you mirror?" If this resistance is particularly strong, one may have to call it out and decide collaboratively with the supervisee about procedures that will counteract this obscurity, such as audio-recording a session or bringing process notes.

Another familiar dynamic in individual supervision that may be relieved by interpretation involves the potentially conflicting narcissistic needs of supervisor and supervisee. Supervisors want to feel useful; they want to have a sense of having added to the supervisee's knowledge and skill. They feel good about themselves when they have offered something, taught something, or enhanced something. Supervisees' narcissistic needs are different. Because of their normal anxiety about being evaluated, their self-esteem depends on hearing the message that they have been a good-enough therapist. Even though they are grateful for practical help, it is easy for them to receive the supervisor's offerings not as gifts but as exposés of all they should have already known and all their failures to have done the "right thing." This mismatch of narcissistic needs can also be dealt with straightforwardly, both by naming it and by the supervisor's taking care not to overwhelm newer clinicians with too many suggestions too soon.

PLAYING WITH ALTERNATIVE SOLUTIONS
TO CLINICAL PROBLEMS

In accord with the overall psychoanalytic ethos or sensibility (McWilliams, 2019), psychodynamic supervision supports the autonomy and potential maturity of the clinician as much as possible. Although there have been psychoanalytic teachers who trained mentees by telling them exactly what to do at each clinical choice point, or relentlessly opined about "standard technique," most of us adopt an open-minded, curious way of talking with supervisees about their options in any clinical situation. We discuss several alternative solutions to a clinical dilemma, trying to predict the probable outcome of each one given our shared understanding of a patient's dynamics, current circumstances, and personal strengths and weaknesses. We emphasize that there are different routes to making the unconscious conscious, that the mentee will eventually find what works best for him or her, and that the ultimate goal of supervision is for supervisees to develop a sense of what is most easily integrated into their own unique style.

As they mature clinically, supervisees may voluntarily seek to learn specific dynamic approaches, such as control–mastery therapy (Silberschatz, 2005), transference-focused psychotherapy (Caligor et al., 2018), mentalization-based therapy (Bateman & Fonagy, 2013), the conversational model (Meares, 2012a, 2012b), dynamic deconstructive psychotherapy (Gregory & Remen, 2008), intensive short-term dynamic psychotherapy (Abbass, 2016), or accelerated experiential dynamic psychotherapy (Fosha, 2005). Or they may want to learn emotion-focused psychotherapy (Greenberg, 2014), a close relative of psychoanalysis, or therapies that can be used adjunctively with analytic work, such as EMDR (Shapiro & Forrest, 1997) or somatic treatments (e.g., Levine & Frederick, 1997; Ogden, Pain, & Minton, 2006). At that point, they will be eager to learn a prescribed protocol and will readily enter an implicit contract to be critiqued on how closely they approximate it. But early in their training, or in the absence of their having chosen to learn a focused model, they need more general nurturing of their capacity to be a healing presence and an appreciation of the fact that there are many different ways to arrive at a therapeutic destination.

Consider, for example, a young woman in supervision who has presented the case of a man whose intimate relationships are burdened by his need to be right. Since that tendency appears in the clinical hour (by his insistence, for instance, that he always knows better than the therapist about whatever they are talking about), how should the therapist respond? She could confront the defense by interpreting the fact that he seems to have learned to attach his self-esteem to a putative infallibility, which may be causing some of his interpersonal problems. That response could be right and yet so narcissistically wounding that the confrontation might be rejected out of hand. Would it be better to tease him gently about the pattern ("You seem to know more than I do about everything!")? Or should she try to disarm him by smiling and saying something like "I knew you'd be correcting me if I said that!"? Or should she try to go *under* the know-it-all defense to the feelings she thinks it is protecting him against ("I thought I saw a look of pain on your face before you corrected me. What's that about?")? Or should she simply absorb this behavior because she feels he is not ready yet to admit to his compulsive, off-putting tendency? Sometimes a supervisee will come up with therapeutic responses that are better than anything the supervisor had been considering.

In clinical situations like this one, I might talk about ways I think I would behave in the session, but with some careful attention to whether my supervisee would find my approach compatible with his or her general stance, and with some reflection on whether my solution would have succeeded or failed. I might note any parallel process phenomena, for example, if my supervisee has an uncharacteristically confident tone that sounds a bit like the patient and affects me the way the patient's tone affects the supervisee. I would expect that my less experienced colleague and I would discuss together not only the patient's probable response to an intervention, but also whether the supervisee could authentically make such an intervention. The key psychoanalytic principle of multiple function (Waelder, 1936) suggests that given the "overdetermination" of any problem important enough to bring a patient to treatment, there are many different directions from which one can intervene (Pine, 2020).

I remember once suggesting to a therapist that he say to a self-defeating patient, "There must be something you're getting out of this tendency to abase yourself." He responded, "*You* could probably get away with saying that, but if *I* did, I'd feel I was blaming the victim, and she'd be likely to accuse me of mansplaining." He proposed that instead he could say, "It's interesting. You seem to be wanting to change this self-destructive pattern, but at the same time, it seems almost automatic. What do you make of that?" Another participant in the consultation group in which this issue came up commented that she might say, "How come I find myself very anxious about your behavior, and yet you seem to have no anxiety at all about it?"

In conversations about the pros and cons of various interventions, it is often valuable for the supervisee to role-play the patient and watch the supervisor struggle over how to respond. Experiencing the client's tone firsthand is basic to the supervisor's emerging understanding of what is going on clinically. With the emotions, tone, and prosody that come through in a role play, new possibilities for interaction may emerge not only for the content of the intervention, but also for the style. A clinician may have all the right words, but if the patient can seize on something in the tone of an observation that feels contemptuous, naïve, or otherwise off base, the "right" words will likely fail to help. Role-playing gives the supervisor a chance to model a tone that might be therapeutic. In the next chapter, I talk at more length about the value of role play in supervision.

One final observation, relevant to colleagues who emphasize inter-subjectivity: Not all supervisee errors are countertransferential—a point made at least as early as 1955 by Annie Reich (Sloane, 1957). Less experienced therapists need information and the wisdom of seasoned teachers as much as they need attention to the thoughts and feelings they bring to any clinical situation. They may have misunderstood the client diagnostically, or have been insensitive to some cultural issue they had no reason to know about, or said something that came from unproblematic intentions but encountered a previously unknown traumatic sensitivity in the patient. When mentors take the implicit or explicit position that the main topic for discussion is the student's subjectivity, they may deprive the clinician of other useful knowledge and, especially with beginning therapists, risk triggering a level of self-consciousness that can interfere with therapeutic effectiveness.

SUPPORTING ETHICAL SENSIBILITIES

Supervisors must hold supervisees accountable for knowing the ethical standards of their profession and the laws that apply to practice (Alonso, 1985). Their specific role is noting when and how these general guidelines apply to here-and-now clinical situations. Not all ethical problems that arise in psychotherapy, however, are resolvable by reference to legal regulations, ethics codes, manuals, or research on relevant topics. As Carol Gilligan's work (e.g., 1982) has demonstrated, there is more than one kind of moral sensibility, and sometimes alternative perspectives on ethical choices are in tension. Most ethical decisions involve evaluating competing moral claims, not finding the only unambiguously correct position.

Consequently, even seasoned therapists seek consultation with colleagues when trying to figure out the right thing to do in a complicated or particularly worrisome clinical situation, such as a patient's flirtation with suicidal wishes or a tendency to scapegoat a child. Such consultation is sensible on its own merits given that we all have blind spots that a colleague can help us look into. It is also good risk management: When clients lodge official complaints against psychotherapists, the regulatory groups and boards responsible for overseeing professional behavior give substantial weight to whether the clinician has consulted with a senior colleague about the issue in question.

Most ethical decisions involve a trade-off, not a clear right versus wrong, and many require a careful weighing of possible consequences by at least two minds. Because there could never be a rulebook covering all possibilities, complicated clinical situations depend on the internal moral gyroscopes of both therapist and supervisor, and these sensibilities evolve with clinical experience. An appreciation that ethical codes and professional rules cannot resolve every ethical problem is an important part of clinical maturation. I go into complex clinical problems more deeply in Chapter 6, which includes an extended example of a dilemma faced by a colleague that illustrates how real-life clinical challenges are sometimes not clearly covered by texts, rules, or protocols. In such situations, at least one supervisory consultation would be vital for any practitioner.

ENCOURAGING THERAPY FOR THE THERAPIST

One of the few areas on which virtually all psychoanalytic therapists agree is the value of psychotherapy for the therapist (see McWilliams, 2004, for the rationale behind this consensus). Analytic training institutes require personal analysis, and most psychodynamically oriented clinical programs strongly encourage personal therapy. Consequently, many of our supervisees have been or are in treatment and fully grasp its value. But psychoanalytic supervisors may also mentor people who do not share this perspective and who feel no inclination to go into therapy unless they are suffering from a diagnosable disorder. Sometimes a newer therapist's undergraduate professor has taken the position that mental health treatments apply only to official DSM categories and are suspect when undertaken with the goal of personal growth. We may believe that some colleagues and potential colleagues could benefit both personally and professionally from their own treatment and yet consider them adequate clinicians. However, we may feel an urgency to get other colleagues to a therapist because their personal dynamics seem to be regularly interfering with their clinical effectiveness.

For example, one early supervisee of mine was deeply identified with the client-centered humanistic tradition. She did well with patients who blossomed under the care of a comforting, sympathetic clinician. But with clients who were notably personality disordered, defensive, or oppositional, she was quite ineffective. They tended to exploit her generosity, which reinforced their problematic dynamics of entitlement and manipulation. They also tended to quit after a few sessions. When I would encourage her to set reasonable limits with a patient, she would protest that I was being "unempathic." This objection applied even to her implementing clinic policies, such as charging patients who had made appointments but who had neglected either to show up or to cancel.

This therapist failed to understand that in her zeal to be a paragon of Rogerian empathy, she was unable, because of her own defenses against noticing anything negative in herself, to empathize with patients' more competitive, hostile, aggressive, and selfish motives. For her, empathy meant identification only with the nicer, needier parts of other people. I had no evidence that she was doing active damage to her clients, but at the same time, she had a disproportionate number of dropouts and was failing to help many of those who needed help the most.

It took me 2 years to talk this supervisee into seeing a therapist. She was highly resistant to the idea, buttressing her position with protestations that she was clinically a "natural," to whom friends and family members had always came with their problems, and that in her Eastern European community of origin there were ample nonprofessional sources of help if she should need it. She implied, in a voice suffused with sympathetic understanding, that my feeling that therapy would be of value to her might simply reflect a knee-jerk adherence to unproven psychoanalytic dogma (this resistance did make me bristle since for some time there has been considerable empirical evidence that therapy has value for the therapist; see Geller et al., 2005). It took one serious depression and several bad experiences with patients—including one who ended up stiffing her on a huge bill that she had let him accumulate without complaint—before she was willing to consider treatment for herself.

It is dicey to suggest therapy to people like this supervisee, who take such suggestions as a criticism of their overall mental health (which, in this instance, it was, though not to the degree she seemed to fear). The main way I try to reduce resistances to personal treatment is by talking about how valuable my own analytic experiences have been to my clinical work. I make that general point, as most analysts would probably do, but in addition, I look for opportunities to "pursue the particular" (Levenson, 1988), to recount specific times when what I learned in treatment helped me with a difficult clinical situation. Sometimes a conversation about what the supervisee is afraid of is useful, but as it verges on therapy rather than supervision, I am reluctant to go there. I do, however, raise questions about how clinicians can sincerely value a service that they devalue when it applies to themselves, and how can they be confident in their helpfulness as a clinician if they have not felt the positive consequences of psychotherapy firsthand.

GRATIFICATIONS OF INDIVIDUAL SUPERVISION AND CONSULTATION

Except for situations in which a supervisee or colleague seeking consultation seems to have serious personality pathology or in which there is a fundamental mismatch between supervisor and supervisee, a problem I address in Chapter 9, most experienced therapists I know say that one-on-one supervision can be both more directly rewarding and easier than individual therapy. The satisfactions are similar to those of any teaching role: One witnesses students' increasing confidence and expertise and feels a parental kind of pride in their accomplishments. Unlike their patients, supervisees rarely have the intrusive, primitive dynamics that make clinical work so demanding; also unlike most patients, they often express straightforward appreciation for our help, leaving our self-esteem more intact than it typically is after sessions with clients.

As for being easier, supervisors hear the therapy process at one remove from the affective intensity of the clinical encounter. Consequently, they may have a better sense of perspective and more objectivity than the supervisee can have. This is a situational phenomenon; it occurs irrespective of the therapist's level of clinical sophistication. Recurrent dynamics are more readily seen at a distance, and the patient's progress is more visible as well. Because supervisors tend to hear about each of the supervisee's clients less frequently than the therapist meets with them, they can more easily see the "forest" of the work and are less distracted by the individual trees. Like the visiting grandparent who exclaims, "My, how you've grown!" when the child's parents have witnessed the evolution too gradually to be struck by it, the supervisor can often see clear progress where the supervisee feels only a slog. Speaking of analogies to family life, I have noticed that both psychotherapy and supervision are often implicitly compared to parenthood. There is an old saw to the effect that the main job of parents is to make themselves unnecessary. The same applies to supervision. The gratifications are similar as well, as one's supervisees become independent centers of professional skill and judgment.

CONCLUDING COMMENTS

In this chapter I have elaborated on some general elements of establishing and strengthening the supervisory alliance and conducting individual supervision. I have emphasized the importance of agreeing on the supervisory contract, formulating realistic and individualized goals for each patient, encouraging frank and open discussion, dealing with resistances to learning, engaging in mutual discussion of alternative possibilities for therapeutic intervention, and supporting each supervisee's maturation as an ethical thinker. Finally, I have summarized some of the gratifications of being a supervisor. Most of these considerations apply also to supervision in group settings, which is the topic of the next chapter.

Chapter Five

■   ■   ■   ■

Group Supervision and Consultation

Consulting in a small-group setting is my favorite mode of supervision, mainly because I learn as much as I teach. As I mentioned in Chapter 1, the most valuable clinical education I ever received was in a counter-transference-focused group in New York City led by Arthur Robbins (see, e.g., 1988). Participation in this intensive experience expanded my knowledge, kept me honest about my struggles and blind spots with patients, reduced the loneliness endemic to private practice, and extended my range as a therapist via the opportunity to identify with other professionals. At a time when my finances were tight, the fact that it was also less expensive than individual supervision was an important consideration, which is a concern for many of the therapists with whom I now consult. Once I got my license, I wanted to offer this experience to colleagues: a variant of peer supervision but with a facilitator who would manage scheduling and other general structural matters, address group-process issues, and contribute relevant expertise.

The chief purpose of a supervision group is to increase the therapeutic skills of members. But it also offers additional benefits in friendship, networking, sharing information on professional issues, and learning for its own sake. It provides a rare sanctuary where therapists can let their hair down, kvetch, laugh, compare experiences, and find consolation. Many clinicians have commented that the existence of one of my groups has helped them to contain intense and troubling countertransferences in the clinical moment, knowing they can vent later to a sympathetic audience. With their colleagues in a group, they can also build on their strengths, improve their facility in giving feedback, develop their own supervisory style, and develop a realistic appreciation of their capacity to make helpful contributions. More than one participant has made a comment like "In this group I've found my own voice."

As of this writing, I lead three private groups composed of six to eight therapists of varying experience, theoretical orientations, and disciplines (psychology; psychiatry; social work; counseling; psychoanalysis; and art, drama, and movement therapies). The newest group began in 1997; the oldest goes back to the late 1970s. Although most members refer to them as supervision groups, they are technically consultation groups, in that the treating therapist retains legal responsibility for the patients presented. Some participants have been in their group for decades. We meet every 2 weeks for 90 minutes to talk about cases, usually taking summers off. Gradually, membership has become predominantly female, perhaps reflecting the feminization of psychotherapy as a field or the greater disposition of women to continue their professional education after licensure or certification, or both.

In addition, since 1982, I have led a fourth group for advanced doctoral candidates at the Graduate School of Applied and Professional Psychology at Rutgers University. Participants have individual supervisors who oversee their cases and are ultimately responsible for the patients they treat and may present in the group. I support their individual supervision, while trying to give students the opportunity to hear a range of perspectives on any clinical and professional development problems they face. The group also provides a place for members to refine their capacity to give supervisory feedback to peers and to notice the growth over time in their general skill level and sense of competence in conceptualizing and commenting on clinical issues.

In the Rutgers group, I attempt to keep membership limited to nine participants, but to make the experience available to all interested students before they graduate, I have sometimes admitted as many as 12 people. In the 2020–2021 academic year, financial pressures on the university related to the COVID-19 pandemic required professors to admit more students than we typically would, and so as I write this, my Rutgers group, with whom I am now meeting weekly on Zoom, has 14 members. This number of participants feels to me and to them too high to make the group feel intimate, but we are trying to make the experience valuable despite that limitation. We meet weekly during the academic year for an hour and a quarter. Usually the group, which the university offers as a one-credit course for advanced students, becomes available in the

third year of their graduate work. Once admitted, participants may stay
as long as they wish. An occasional student has remained for 3 or 4
years, but there is significant turnover annually as people graduate or
leave for internships.

OVERVIEW

In all my groups, the participating therapists present their cases, especially challenging ones, with the exception of those involving anyone they
know to be recognizable to me or another member. In the rare instance
when a student unexpectedly recognizes the patient being presented, he
or she exits the group for that day. At the beginning of the semester in
the Rutgers group, I ask students to inform me privately if they know
any of my own patients or supervisees, so that I can avoid using that
individual's personal or clinical material to illustrate some point I want
to make. In the other groups, I simply remind members periodically to
tell me in confidence if they learn that someone they know is in treatment or supervision with me.

In one of my groups, the participating therapists eventually decided
to take turns presenting in a regular order, alphabetically by the last
name of the member, but the convention is suspended if one of them is
facing a clinical crisis. The other groups follow the principle of "Whoever needs the time claims it." Discussions of professional matters are
welcome (e.g., cancellation policies, issues of payment, insurance headaches, legal and ethical issues, resources for patients with particular
needs, upcoming conferences), as are observations on group process. I
ask participants to voice any concerns about how the group is going and
to mention in particular any dynamics that interfere with their comfort
in describing their work.

The role requirement of a member of a supervision group is to
attend regularly, to talk as honestly as possible about the transactions
between themselves and their clients, to be considerate of other members' feelings and needs, to be sensitive to the ethical complexities of
talking about patients, and to try to bring up any issue that seems to
be getting in the way of people's sense of safety and comfort presenting
their clinical work. Relatively quiet participants are as valued as those
who speak frequently. Despite the invitation for members to raise any
sense of resistance to the task at hand, I rarely have to deal with group-
process issues. Participants, many of whom, even in the student group,
have better training in group dynamics than I do, are generally alert

to the manifestations of common themes such as competition, feelings of being criticized, ambivalence toward new members, reactions to the loss of a member, and unfinished emotional business from the previous meeting. They are usually quick to address any impediments to a sense of safety, but if I sense that a problem in that area is haunting a group's smooth functioning, I contribute my impression.

At their best, supervision groups provide a deeply intimate, emotionally satisfying kind of learning. Members reveal their most painful misunderstandings and mistakes so that they can understand them, rectify them if possible, and avoid repeating them. At their worst, groups can be traumatizing. Members can feel painfully exposed, to the point of unbearable humiliation and emotional shutdown. Early in my training I once felt emotionally violated by a group leader, an experience that needlessly delayed my progress in trusting others with my innermost thoughts. It would be hard to overestimate the vulnerability felt by therapists, especially newer therapists, when describing their work to peers, a situation in which they feel at risk of group shaming.

My group-supervision experience with Arthur Robbins was profoundly self-exposing and consistently positive because of the atmosphere of safety he engendered, but when I started leading groups for colleagues, I knew that his rather penetrating style was a bad fit with my own personality. I could not have adopted his approach authentically or in a way that would reliably avoid hurting people. In addition, the context of my work was different from his. Most people in his groups attend them after years of psychoanalytic immersion as patients and students. They expect to explore the nooks and crannies of their own psyches, sometimes encountering strong emotions in the process. In contrast, my groups seem to appeal to many clinicians *without* much psychodynamic background. Frequently, therapists seek them out to add psychoanalytic ideas, especially psychoanalytic knowledge about personality differences, to their clinical repertoire. They have not signed up to bare their souls and would probably feel invaded and exposed if I were to probe into their dynamics.

In reflecting on my work as a leader over the years with groups for clinicians, I have concluded that I serve four basic functions. First, members expect me to provide knowledge: to speak as a seasoned practitioner and to refer them to literature or resources that can illuminate and guide their work with a particular client. Second, they rely on me for housekeeping tasks. They need me to keep track of the schedule, to remember whose turn it is to present, to decide whether or not to cancel in bad weather, to interview potential new members, to arrange for flowers to be sent to a participant who has lost a loved one, and so on.

Third, they rely on me to slow things down and protect the presenter from feeling overwhelmed when feedback is coming too fast or is interrupting too often to allow adequate space for reflection. Finally, when they have identified a group dynamic that interferes with their freedom to learn, they look to me for leadership in resolving it. Each group has its own "personality," and each seems to have different preferences as to how much of each function is called for.

The student group has distinctive sensibilities. Its overall group personality varies from year to year, but some general themes have recurred over my tenure as group leader. Let me now share some observations about the student group and about issues specific to group supervision in the context of a training program. I assume that my observations could be adapted to educational settings that include medical residency, master's and doctoral programs, and postgraduate training institutes. In all these situations, the fact that one is being evaluated for one's readiness to occupy a more independent or expert role both catalyzes and complicates the learning process.

GROUP SUPERVISION WITH THERAPISTS IN TRAINING

In my group at Rutgers, students take turns as needed presenting difficult cases. Sometimes they compare notes on shared problems. Their activity might include expressing anxieties about potentially suicidal patients; making efforts to understand the inner world of clients from significantly different cultural and religious backgrounds; voicing the pain of absorbing micro- (and not so micro-) aggressions based on the student's race, age, accent, or appearance; condoling about the tortures of internship applications (including the pain of competing for placements with other group members who have previously been in mostly supportive roles); articulating the misery of having to terminate with a patient who is not ready to stop therapy; managing psychotherapy that involves ancillary treatments (e.g., twelve-step programs, EMDR, psychiatric consultation, DBT groups); sharing the challenges of dealing with family members and third parties; and sympathetically sharing the pressures they feel from administrators in their clinical placements. More rarely, a presenter will talk about a problem with a supervisor and ask for the group's suggestions about how to bring that issue up tactfully in the person's individual supervision.

Sometimes a group member describes a supervisory or consultation experience that strikes others as damaging, unprofessional, or simply a distraction from the supervisory task, and we brainstorm about how the student can deal with the situation. For example, one female group member was working with an older male supervisor who had a young adult daughter about whom he was worried. He was consistently using the woman's supervision time to query her about the sexual conventions of her generation. Assuming she was heterosexual (when, in fact, she was more fluid but reluctant to say so because of his evident prejudices), he implicitly kept asking her to "other" those in her age cohort whose sexuality was less binary than he felt proper. Because of his improper use of her time with him in these self-serving ways, her learning about how to help her patients consistently got short shrift. Learning how to extract the best from any mentor and how to keep supervisors on task, whatever their idiosyncrasies, is a developmental challenge with which a peer group can be quite helpful. In addition, I have found that student group members collectively are also pretty good judges of when one should look into the possibility of working with a different supervisor.

The group provides a secure base and a safe space to compare stresses and disillusionments. As our overall mental health system in the United States suffers increasingly severe pressures to cut costs, student complaints of feeling patronized by overworked and distracted staff members in the agencies where they have practicum assignments or internship positions are increasingly common. Graduate students are held to high legal and ethical standards at Rutgers, and they are sometimes upset to witness the extent to which those standards are ignored in many contemporary training sites, which are typically overburdened, understaffed, subject to high turnover, and governed by bureaucrats far from the front lines of clinical service. I hear many reports about authorities who care more about whether a discharge form was filled out than whether the discharge summary makes any psychological sense or would be helpful to future clinicians treating the patient who is being discharged.

Because participants in the Rutgers group are burdened with the status of students under evaluation, there seems to be a greater need there for me to address issues such as competition for my approval, insider–outsider themes (often presenting as old member–new member rivalries), and inhibitions about expressing negative reactions to things I might say. At the same time, graduate-student groups are particularly hungry for content. Consequently, I find that striking a balance between providing knowledge and processing dynamics is harder in that group than in others I lead. Often the tension between wishes to be taught and wishes to discuss group issues in a more participatory way manifests itself as a split between those who ask me to speak more conceptually about the case being presented and those who want to explore the interpersonal currents in the group so as to find meaning there.

I remember in this context a time when a male student was presenting a heterosexual female patient with a strikingly self-defeating pattern. The client for whom he had originally felt deep compassion now struck him as a whining complainer and, as a result, the presenter's countertransference had become painfully negative. The woman repeatedly expressed a need for his advice on how to live less dangerously, but whenever he suggested that she consider an alternative option, she would dismiss it. For example, she was in the habit of having unprotected sex with strangers she picked up in bars, but she would respond to the therapist's questions about whether she had used a condom, or whether she had asked anything about the man's sexual history, with reassurances that although she had not, the guy "seemed clean" and had struck her as "nice enough." (This is a common phenomenon with self-defeating patients; they may have a genius for putting anxiety about their self-destructiveness into the therapist and then evidently thinking that because the therapist is on the case, they now do not have to reflect on what they are doing; see McWilliams, 2011, chap. 12.)

About half the students in the group wanted to talk about their own emotional reactions to the presentation. They found themselves quite disturbed to be feeling so internally condemnatory of a client who had had a terrible history and was clearly suffering. They felt she was torturing the therapist, and they were experiencing a kind of secondary torment. The remaining members wanted me to talk about masochism in general and about how to understand cognitively the meaning of self-defeating patterns. Because the presenter wanted more conceptual support from me, I talked more about the latter, but I also generalized about the hateful and even sadistic feelings one can have for patients with characterological tendencies toward bad judgment and self-destructive actions.

In the Rutgers group, I rarely know much about the personal attachments of students to one another. They may have intense and complicated relationships outside the group setting that have an inhibiting effect on what they say. In this situation, presenters may have to bring up relational dynamics that are patent to them but invisible to me. Especially because graduate students typically idealize mentors and thus imagine that my intuition goes beyond clinical areas, they are surprised that their interpersonal dynamics are not more obvious to me. In such situations of inhibition due to the dynamics external to the group, an appreciation of the unequal status of the student and faculty member leads me to be careful not to push participants beyond their comfort level for exposure.

When initially orienting students to group norms, I ask that they scrupulously avoid talking outside the group about what goes on inside it, thus protecting the privacy not only of the patients presented, but also of any classmate who reveals something personally intimate.

I express my belief that it is highly beneficial to the group process when members feel safe enough to divulge their own histories, problems, and dynamics, but I note that different groups develop different norms each year about how much members are comfortable sharing. I state explicitly that I will try not to "pull" for intimate material, as I know very little about the relationships of the people in the group and have no idea how safe it is for them to speak unguardedly. Thus, my official position is that I welcome self-disclosure, but only when it comes voluntarily from the student. I try to remind members periodically that if I ask a question that a person experiences as too intrusive, he or she should say so and decline to go there.

That said, I occasionally have had to protect a member who I thought was being self-disclosing in a way that felt emotionally self-endangering or overstimulating to others. In such instances, I might steer the group toward a change of topic and/or invite the student to talk with me privately after the meeting. Once, for example, a woman with a significant trauma history, who was understandably reactive to descriptions of patients with childhood sexual abuse, began to recount, in a slightly dissociated tone, graphic details of her early molestation. Because I feared she was retraumatizing herself and also at risk of being seen by others as too fragile to bear certain clinical topics that come up frequently, I gently interrupted her account and reoriented the conversation. I talked to her afterward about what I saw as the difference between, on one hand, noting that one has a trauma history and thus has firsthand wisdom that can help clinicians with traumatized patients and, on the other hand, bringing specific traumatic experiences so vividly into listeners' imaginations that defensive distancing would be the expectable consequence.

As I stated in Chapter 1, in the Rutgers group, my own efforts to accept criticism without defensiveness seem particularly vital to participants' professional maturation. Students report that they are relieved to learn that speaking the truth to an individual with power is not necessarily dangerous, and that therapeutic authorities can admit to and apologize for mistakes. Many years ago, for example, when I was excited about having learned some hypnotic techniques that can help patients who dissociate find an internal place of safety, I rashly suggested that a student presenter do some hypnotic work with his client. When he protested that he had no training in hypnosis, I told him it was easy to learn and proceeded to describe how to evoke a light trance in a cooperative patient. At the next meeting, he criticized me, and his classmates joined in. One reported having said to him, "You're not gonna *take* that crazy advice, are you?" I apologized, asking for their sympathetic understanding of my excessive enthusiasm for a newly acquired technique, and I made clear my regret at having casually urged them to go beyond both their skill levels and their comfort zones.

Although they are more dramatically evident in the context of working with students, blundering and copping to blundering may be critical therapeutic processes for any leader. As analytic writers have long pointed out (e.g., Casement, 1985, 2002; Fors, 2018; Kohut, 1977; Maroda, 1991, 1999; Wolf, 1988), the therapeutic effect when a person with power admits to and explores the effects of an empathic failure can be worth the pain of the mistake. Therapists, especially those in training, tend to have perfectionistic defenses that are reinforced by regular admonitions about appropriate behavior and professional responsibility. They need exemplars who can keep their self-esteem despite acknowledged limitations and mistakes. They also need to take in the unwelcome but ultimately liberating fact that just as no physician can cure every patient and no teacher can make a scholar out of every student, no therapist, no matter how good one's intentions and one's training, succeeds in helping every patient.

PRAGMATICS OF GROUP SUPERVISION

In a typical supervision/consultation group meeting, one participant presents a patient in detail, although sometimes, if two therapists have a pressing clinical issue, they split the time. Although they may bring notes about the patient's background, presenters speak spontaneously rather than from carefully prepared material, which tends to mute the affective tone and spontaneous bodily expression that are vital to clinical understanding. Group members expect presenters to begin by mentioning the general nature of the problem they are trying to solve, so that they can focus in on that issue. Perhaps, for example, the presenter feels the treatment is stalled by some stubborn resistance. Perhaps the therapist cannot find a way into a cognitive understanding or empathic feeling for the patient. Perhaps he or she has fallen into in an intense countertransference or worrisome enactment. After noting their main concerns, presenters then report the client's overall demographics: age, relationship status, gender identification and sexual orientation, ethnic and cultural background, religious identification, socioeconomic position, occupation, and so on.

Then they note how long and at what frequency they have seen the patient, what he or she originally came to therapy for, what the history of the presenting complaint is, and whether the patient has had prior treatment. It helps the group if presenters bring the client to life with descriptions of the individual's general physical presentation, verbal style, body language, and inferred attitude toward the therapist. Finally, they summarize the client's history, with an emphasis on family members and caregivers both objectively (age; health status or deceased; occupation; any known diagnoses) and subjectively (how the client experienced them and described their personalities). Presenters often speculate on the client's attachment style. Some like to pass out genograms. Occasionally they mention psychological or neurological testing. Moves, losses, illnesses, injuries, and stressful or traumatic experiences are reported. Earliest memories, recurrent dreams, and illuminating childhood stories might be part of the presentation as well, and, if presenters have the patient's permission, they will occasionally share artwork, poetry, or journal entries with the group. Sometimes they will read email threads or texts.

This summary ordinarily takes about half an hour. The group members listen, mostly quietly, to the presenter's clinical situation, trying to grasp the overall psychology of the client and how it infuses the relationship with the therapist. They usually ask questions to clarify or expand on areas about which they find themselves confused or ignorant. Eventually they offer feedback that includes hypotheses about case formulation, resistance, transference, and countertransference. They also give moral support, associate to comparable clinical experiences, and suggest interventions. Often, most fruitfully, they report their emotional reactions, with the shared assumption that they are a revealing parallel to what is going on between client and therapist (Ekstein & Wallerstein, 1958/1971). After this process, I tend to join the conversation with thoughts about the client's personality, maturational course, and other features that might help with the problem being addressed. If I know about literature that illuminates an issue that seems central to understanding the person and the treatment, I recommend it or send them an article after the meeting.

When a presentation seems stilted or intellectualized, I might encourage the presenter to role-play the client, while I or another group member tries to act as therapist. Any doubts people have about the inevitability of introjection, the process whereby others get into our head and register their presence in our less conscious mental realms, will be dispelled by role play. It is remarkable how quickly the presenter "becomes" the client, and how much more clearly the observers can then comprehend what the therapist has been dealing with. Role-playing permits the affective tone of the work to be more present without the presenter's having to accept sole responsibility for the countertransference.

Frequently, when I have role-played the therapist while the presenting clinician role-plays the client, I have approached the interaction with confidence that I know a way to dissolve the clinical stalemate. But then I find myself immediately in the same emotional quagmire from which the presenter has been trying to get extricated. At this point I give voice to all my ugly feelings and fantasies before trying to solve the problem of technique. This is comforting to both the presenter and the group members. I remember a recent presentation in which I thought it would be easy to get a patient moving in a therapeutic direction. When I role-played the therapist, however, all my clever moves were brilliantly thwarted. "I hate this patient!" I found myself shouting. After this catharsis, we all managed to figure out a promising strategy to take the work in a better direction.

A common experience in consultation groups is that participants find themselves in touch with feelings that the presenting clinician has disowned or unconsciously ignored. Several times I have heard a group member lovingly present a patient with an erotic transference. The presenter has decided to talk about this person because something feels disturbing about the countertransference attraction to the patient or because the therapist knows that sexually charged clinical situations should be discussed with colleagues before they go down a slippery slope (Celenza, 2011; Gabbard, 2016). The clinician tends to be focused on the client's charming qualities, whereas the group fails to see what is so attractive about the person. Members typically find themselves disliking the client, whom they experience as using seductiveness in the service of undermining their colleague's proper role and winning a power struggle seen only by the client. The presenter tends to protest this perception at first, creating a dichotomy between presenter and group.

At this point, I tend to intervene with an empathic description of the patient's feeling of weakness and defensive use of sexuality to turn the tables on an authority whom he or she fears. In other words, I try to model compassion coexisting with an awareness of the hostile power play inherent in sexualized efforts to dominate the clinician. After this kind of presentation, the smitten therapist often feels released from the grip of countertransference infatuation. Thus relieved and confident in the boundaries again, he or she can proceed to address tactfully the fear and hostility behind the patient's seductiveness, while not shaming the person for the normal wish to be seen as attractive.

Humor and playfulness are somehow easier in a group setting. The increased interpersonal space creates what contemporary analysts call a "third" (Benjamin, 2017), that is, an expansion that reduces the probability of polarized good-versus-bad experiences. The enjoyment of shared jokes and in-group lore is part of what attracts clinicians to group supervision. Mistakes, limitations, and miserable countertransferences that are mutually acknowledged and laughed about can feel very different from one's experience when an individual supervisor jokes about one's clinical errors. Certain patients, presented recurrently, become famous in a consultation group for qualities such as devaluation, passivity, or aggressiveness. With humor, group members can help the presenter tolerate working patiently with such people and can witness their progress over time.

Toward the end of each group meeting, I try to remember to ask the presenter whether the advice that the rest of us offered was helpful. It gives that person a chance to acknowledge the useful contributions of others and to let us know what was less valuable or where the therapist continues to feel stuck. Such queries also offer an opportunity for the presenter to express any lingering sense of being criticized or misunderstood, along with any remaining discomfort over the self-exposure that goes with describing one's work. Usually, I am slightly surprised at what the presenting clinician emphasizes as the most helpful elements of the conversation. Once, for example, a presenter said, "It was great. That joke Mary made was the highlight." Idiosyncratic differences between one clinician and another tend to underscore the point that in determining a clinical direction, we have to think about each person's unique sensibilities.

SUPERVISION IN GROUPS OF TWO

I have occasionally worked with two therapists who share an hour or more of my supervisory time. My husband, Michael Garrett, supervises hospital residents in pairs on a regular basis. Both of us originally decided on this arrangement for the sake of economies of time and/or money, but we learned that tandem supervision or consultation has some distinctive advantages that may be particularly applicable to therapists in training. It can be valuable for them to realize that their peers struggle as they do, and in instances in which the supervisor praises the work of their colleague, they can get the message that good work is within their grasp. When feedback is more negative, they can see that they are not the only ones who screw up.

In larger groups, some members can be very quiet, but in dyads, participants cannot hide. The listening process is inherently active. At any moment, the supervisor may turn to the person who is not presenting and ask for the nonpresenter's take on the patient or the clinical interaction. This reality encourages the nonpresenter to think deeply about a case and to note the fantasies and images that come to mind. A back-and-forth conversation reduces the pressure on the presenter, who has periods to relax and find out what the other therapist is thinking. If the supervisor is respectful and avoids shaming, it allows the two participants to lament the challenges of the work without having the more daunting exposure to a class or cohort.

The performance dimension of presenting to a supervisor with a colleague in attendance can create a mutual playfulness, lightening an atmosphere otherwise darkened by the grim details of a patient's suffering and the challenges it has created for those trying to help the person. As therapists present their work over time to each other and to the supervisor, the long-term follow-up time for each patient is essentially doubled by the participation of the peer.

RESISTANCES AND COMPLICATIONS
IN SUPERVISION AND CONSULTATION GROUPS

There is a recurrent tension in supervision or consultation groups between wishes for cognitive mastery and wishes to express and explore the complicated affects that the client and/or group process evokes. Although the contract in such groups does not involve treatment, the in-depth learning that may transpire there has therapeutic effects, and some members explicitly pursue them. Sometimes the tension between the intellectual and emotional levels of discourse is embodied by different group members. One person complains, "We stay too much in our heads," and urges deeper exploration of personal countertransferences, while another wants me to "teach more." At other times, this dynamic emerges as a shared group ambivalence. Members become aware of both wanting and not wanting to expose the dynamics in themselves that have become activated by a patient's psychotherapy.

As with student groups, I address such tensions proactively. I state that I try to foster an atmosphere in which emotional intimacy will evolve organically over time, potentiating the right-brain to right-brain processes that make for deeper learning (Schore, 2016). But I emphasize as well that I respect individual differences in willingness to disclose. To encourage self-revelation without intruding on members' privacy, I express my own feelings frequently, associating to clients who have activated my own particular dynamics, bemoaning the affective stresses of the work, and naming the emotions that a clinical portrayal is evoking. I may also associate to personal experiences, both clinical and nonclinical, mention songs that are going through my head, or share images or phrases that pop into my mind.

Having been trained to listen "with the third ear" (Reik, 1948) to how the patient's material stimulates my inner associations, I try to expose my own primary-process reactions. In recent years, recollections of my grandchildren's antics seem to arise a lot when I listen to case presentations, especially those of individuals whose mental processes are on the more primitive side. For example, once when a group member was presenting a person who was masterful at projecting and displacing his less-than-stellar qualities onto others (e.g., "It was my boss's fault. If he hadn't been so hostile, I would've been happy to comply"), I found myself associating to the imaginary friend of my then 5-year-old grandson, who attributed to "Ghosty" any mistake he made or prurient interest he had (especially in farting, it would seem).

Supervisory tact is particularly critical in a group setting. In individual supervision, if I hurt a therapist's feelings, he or she can react to me in private. Hurt feelings are more painful when witnessed by an audience. Anxieties about presenting one's work are somewhat different in individual and group situations, respectively. Although in both settings the presenter may be braced for the supervisor's potential disapproval, fears of humiliation tend to be greater in the latter. But at the same time, the group situation allows therapists to witness colleagues' anxieties about the leader's evaluation and to realize that these reactions constitute a more or less universal response to supervision, not a distinctively neurotic problem of their own.

One other advantage of group consultation is that the modeling of nonhumiliating feedback invites supervisees to identify with the leader's efforts to be considerate and kind. Although therapists in training are typically so ready to feel negatively evaluated that they never miss the criticism in even the most tactful comment, they appreciate the attempt to protect their feelings, and they may remember and hold themselves up to the standard of this kind of consideration. In conferring a teaching award to an admired supervisor, Razieh Adabimohazab, then an advanced psychiatric resident in a supervision group for clinicians treating psychotic patients, teased him with the following summary of his style of intervention:

> Some know him with this phrase: "I am going to make a joke now with your permission." Sometimes after one makes a comment in a supervision, there is this short pause and then he goes "Hmm! That too! But also . . . " and that is the moment you find out your comment was completely off the topic. Thanks for teaching us how to feel comfortable sharing our personal stories and our flaws, having in mind there is no judgment or shame in the room. (June 20, 2019, quoted with permission)

In my experience, obvious resistance to supervision in a voluntary group setting is not very common. When it is, it may be manifested by members' absences, repeated lateness, or "not having anything to present." The last situation may not always indicate an unconscious resistance to learning, however. Therapists, who tend to have both characterological and learned tendencies to put the needs of others ahead of their own, may hesitate to present if someone else is seen as "needing the time more." Frequently, group members are amused by the reaction formation with which they handle competitive situations: "You go ahead and present; I presented recently." "No, *you* take the time today; you have a more pressing issue." Although not a particularly serious resistance, this can be an impediment to the natural give-and-take of participation.

As groups mature and members get more clinical experience, there is usually a shift from "I don't know what I'm doing with this client!" to "I guess I could present someone I think I'm working okay with, but whom I'd like to understand better." Sometimes I intervene when I feel a member is being excessively generous and not claiming a fair share of airtime; this habit seems especially characteristic of female participants (see McWilliams & Stein, 1987, for some thoughts about the group effects of women's reluctance to compete). In my group in which members present cases in regular rotation, the participants decided on that arrangement because it had become rare for them to feel a beginner's urgency about getting help.

The more voluntary a person's membership in a group, the fewer resistive dynamics seem to arise. At one time, I had some group members who were accruing hours toward licensure, and I found that they typically had more ambivalence about attending than the other participants did. Interestingly, more than one such member has dropped out upon being licensed, reportedly because the members were simply tired of having been in the student role "forever." In one instance, a woman who had left after passing the New Jersey psychology licensing exam returned 2 years later, commenting that her experience was dramatically different now that supervision was no longer another hoop she had to jump through to attain legitimacy. The sense of ownership of the learning process can thus counteract the inherent discomforts of self-exposure.

Occasionally, a member provokes a difficult group dynamic, but only once in 40-plus years have I had to ask a participant to switch groups because of such a problem (the person did, and the second group was more forgiving of her idiosyncrasies; in fact, they became deeply fond of her over time). Sometimes, a new member will take a personal dislike to me or my style or to a clinician in the group and decide not to continue. This problem occurs infrequently enough that I tend not to notice it happening; recently, a newish member in one of my groups decided to leave on the grounds of feeling unwelcome by the other therapists. In retrospect, I wish I had addressed the member's discomfort before it culminated in a decision to quit, but I was slow to recognize it.

The main limitation of group supervision is that the leader cannot effectively address problems caused by significant personality pathology in a therapist. This is hard enough to do in individual supervision; it is virtually impossible in a group setting. Attention to a participant's psychopathology can provoke extreme defensiveness and create a sense of helpless irritation in a group. I have not found a therapist's severe mental health concerns to be a frequent problem, but it does happen. Possible solutions involve private conversations between the group leader and the problematic member, encouragement of the person to seek treatment if he or she is not already seeing a therapist, a referral to individual supervision with another mentor to be conducted concurrently with group meetings, and, as a last resort, possible removal from the group.

Therapists are highly compassionate about personality problems, but when their group process suffers unduly from one member's psychopathology, participants should not be expected to tolerate the cost to their ongoing learning. They have enough exposure to people with personality pathology in their clinical hours, and they look to the group to relieve them of chronically having to be mindful of the hypersensitivities of others. Although I have found it rare that one has to counsel a professional out of participating in a consultation group, when the group experience of the other members has been compromised by a significantly problematic colleague, to do so feels like an ethical commitment to their continuing education.

LONG-TERM BENEFITS OF SUPERVISION AND CONSULTATION GROUPS

Perhaps the greatest advantage of being in a group for clinicians that is led by a more experienced therapist is that the experience instills in members a sense of comfort with showing their work to colleagues. Participating in a group can lay the groundwork for their doing so throughout their careers. Perhaps more than other orientations, the psychoanalytic tradition has been committed to ongoing self-examination and lifelong attention to countertransference and personal blind spots. We need to expose what we do to colleagues who know what it is like to work in depth with intense transferences and complex clinical challenges. One outcome of the group mode of learning is that it may encourage participants to lead their own groups later in their careers or to establish a regularly meeting peer group in the future.

We have ample clinical lore about the value of peer supervision groups. I know of such groups in New Jersey that have been in existence for decades, whose members are impressively devoted to their weekly or biweekly meetings. Although there is very little scholarly work on the topic, a welcome exception is Lee Kassan's (2010) book, *Peer Supervision Groups: How They Work and Why You Need One*. In a systematic qualitative study, Kassan documented in fascinating detail the benefits of such groups for psychoanalytic practitioners. It is my hope that being in group supervision during one's training can lay the groundwork for this kind of ongoing and deepening support for professional growth.

CONCLUDING COMMENTS

Some of my colleagues, both academic and clinical, have expressed a reluctance to recommend group supervision, especially for beginning therapists. They may feel that students are not ready for this level of exposure, or they may worry that the group model somehow "dilutes" the purer, more powerful paradigm of individual consultation. It is true that there are significant advantages to the one therapist/one supervisor mode. But there are also areas in which the group or tandem model is superior. It permits multiple perspectives, a range of identifications, the relaxation of many anxieties intrinsic to the role of supervisees, and the benefits of feeling less lonely in the inherently isolating role of clinician. It supports the growth of participants toward being good supervisors themselves, giving them multiple models of what to do (and sometimes what not to do) when giving feedback to other clinicians.

Supervising in a group setting can also be more stimulating to the supervisor than mentoring on an individual basis. Even when members are in the earliest stages of training, their varying skill sets, their diverse personal experiences, and the pooling of their knowledge can widely expand a leader's learning and repertoire of therapeutic interventions. And one cannot do supervision in groups without noticing that often the ideas of some less experienced group member are better than one's own. This humbling aspect of the group situation is a beneficial corrective to what may be the worst occupational hazard of a career in individual therapy and supervision, namely, the reinforcement of grandiosity borne of repeated experiences of being idealized and/or treated as very important (see McWilliams, 1987).

As I stated in the previous chapter, I have been impressed over the course of my career with how deep and compelling is the human wish to continue to learn and grow, and especially to feel increasingly personally effective and useful to others. When respect is maximized and shame is minimized in a group setting, the participating professionals usually open themselves eagerly to learning. As they develop as clinicians, there is discernable improvement in their patients. Nothing could be more fortifying of their commitment to group participation. I feel privileged to have witnessed the clinical maturation of so many talented and conscientious practitioners in the context of experiential and educative groups, and I continue to be grateful for the experience.

Chapter Six

■　■　■　■

Supervision and Ethics

THE LARGER CONTEXT

Clinical supervision transcends issues of effectiveness in the consulting room. It inevitably enters the territory of what is morally right: for the patient, the supervisee, and the larger community. In psychoanalytic therapy, we deliberately foster a powerful attachment that stimulates intense wishes and fears. Because we ask patients to trust us with their deepest shame, their darkest secrets, and their worst vulnerabilities to emotional pain, our consequent ethical obligations should weigh heavily on us as both therapists and mentors.

ORIENTING PREMISES

Psychotherapy does not happen in a vacuum. Although clinicians try not to impose their personal beliefs on their clients (e.g., about religious dogma, electoral politics, or personal sexual morality), both therapist and patient operate within the context of societal values that the surrounding culture expects supervisors to represent. As I suggested earlier, a sacred aspect of the supervisory role is passing on to the next generation of practitioners the moral sensibilities that inform psychotherapy. Many philosophically sophisticated scholars view psychotherapy itself as an ethical practice, a perspective most recently and eloquently argued

by Kevin Smith (2021a, 2021b). In addition to this concern about passing on the moral compass of our discipline, mentors and consultants
bear a responsibility to protect the public against clinicians who are disabled, incompetent, or corrupt.

Recent psychoanalytic literature has framed the context within
which therapy happens as a "moral third" (Benjamin, 2017). Similar to
Jean-Jacques Rousseau's famous notion that the social contract "forces
us to be free" (i.e., to be our best selves, making the choices our most
mature sensibilities prefer), therapists' awareness of shared values can
prevent a collapse into dyadic fantasies, such as "You and I are excep-
tional and responsible to no one but ourselves"—a rationalization that
has supported many transgressions. The holding environment of psychotherapy is neither universal nor static; societal claims on therapists
vary from one culture to another and change with sociopolitical evolu-
tions. When I began my career, for example, confidentiality in therapy
was assumed to be absolute, but then the 1976 *Tarasoff* decision initi-
ated a series of exceptions to that inviolability that have gradually had
far-reaching effects on practice (see Bollas & Sundelson, 1995; Furlong,
2005).

In Chapter 1, I emphasized the complexity of the ethical dilemmas that therapists face, the limitations of codes and regulations, the
problem of competing moral perspectives, the importance of developing
clinical wisdom, the need for therapists at all levels of experience to seek
appropriate help with ethical problems, and the value of the supervisor's
demonstrating integrity. I expand on those themes here, focusing first on
supervisory challenges involving the patient's right to know treatment-
relevant information, then on the supervision of clinical choices affecting mostly the patient–therapist relationship, and finally on supervisory
responsibilities to the community. The complexity of the supervisory
context and the idiosyncratic nature of most ethical dilemmas require
elaboration. Thus, I discuss several vignettes in more length than usual.

RESPECTING THE PATIENT'S RIGHT TO KNOW

In more paternalistic days, many health professionals felt entitled to
withhold vital information if they saw nondisclosure as being in the
patient's best interest. Now, most of us would say that many crimes were
rationalized this way; practitioners hid behind this privilege rather than
facing the consequences of delivering bad news. (My own adamancy
on this point doubtless reflects my childhood experiences with doctors

who decided to "protect" my stepmother from knowing she had cancer, a decision with many negative consequences for my family.) In analytic therapies, clinicians have legitimate reasons to be careful about what they disclose, but some information rightfully belongs to the patient.

I have argued elsewhere (Fors & McWilliams, 2016) that therapists should share medical records with patients. There follow some other areas in which I believe it is ethically incumbent upon us to supply clients with information; I have chosen the areas that may be the most taxing to supervisors as they try to further their supervisees' ethical development. I'm sure there are exceptions to many of the positions I take here; ultimately, much comes down to professional judgment, or to what the United States judicial system has sometimes called the judgment of a "reasonable person."

The Therapist's Training and Background

Although beginners are self-conscious about being beginners, patients have a right to know what training their therapist has had. Supervisors can help a lot here by making suggestions for how clinicians might respond to queries about their credentials—for example, "Yes, I'm in training, in my second year. Do you have concerns about that?" Or, if the supervisee feels there is room for playing a bit, "Yes, I'm still in graduate school. Are you worried I'm not experienced enough? If so, let me reassure you that I make up for my inexperience with my determination to help." If a patient of a therapist who is not able to practice independently asks for the supervisor's name, this level of curiosity warrants exploration (probably before answering), but here also, I think the client has a right to know the information, because in this case it is the supervisor who has ultimate responsibility.

Questions for clinicians at any level about their education, postgraduate training, and overall theoretical orientation may be explored but also should be answered. If these questions arise in the middle of a treatment instead of at the beginning, supervisors can suggest to supervisees that they explore their meaning before addressing their content ("I'm happy to answer that question, but first, can you say why it's coming up now for you?"). After talking about any underlying dynamics, sometimes the question fades in importance, and the client drops it. But if the client persists, such queries deserve a reply. If the therapist's responses to questions like these elicit more invasive questioning, at that point the therapist's legitimate privacy should be respected, and the patient's curiosity should be explored instead of gratified.

Information about How Therapy Works

Several decades ago, most middle-class people in Western societies had some sense of the underlying premises of psychoanalytic treatment. You had to come regularly and talk freely, and you expected change to evolve gradually from a collaboration between you and the therapist. In this era of competing approaches, clinicians are frequently asked questions such as "How is this supposed to help?" Psychodynamic therapy is particularly hard for some clients to grasp, especially if they already have been told that they need to be treated with medication or skills training. Supervisors can do a great service to newer clinicians by suggesting ways to depict analytic treatment so that clients can readily understand it. They can also refer supervisees to readable descriptions of psychodynamic therapies that can be found, for example, on the websites of some psychoanalytic training programs. These accounts are often written clearly enough to be shared with nonprofessionals.

Boundary Conditions of the Treatment

One of the commonest mistakes made by supervisors of psychology graduate students is failing to advise them to tell patients entering long-term or open-ended treatments that at the end of their third or fourth year in the program, they will be leaving for internship placements. Neglecting to tell patients about the time limits imposed by training demands can leave them feeling betrayed when such a transition approaches; termination is then miserable for both client and therapist. One or both may have assumed that the treatment was going to be brief, but in contrast to explicitly short-term therapy models that specify a time period or number of sessions, the length of treatment is not predictable at the beginning of an open-ended therapy. In the absence of information about other limits, patients may assume that the therapeutic collaboration can go on indefinitely.

At the other end of the career arc, therapists who know they will be moving or retiring should inform patients about those plans. The right to know as early as possible applies also to vacations, professional trips, and other foreseeable interruptions to treatment. Supervisors give different advice about how to introduce such information. Some suggest that therapists disclose their plans at the beginning of a session so that patients have time to express and explore their reactions. But because this process can preempt issues the patient was expecting to talk about, and because patients frequently have a delayed response anyway, I tend to advise that therapists bring up this information toward the end of the session and then listen for its effects in the following meeting. This choice about the timing of such disclosures is one of many that has no right answer and may need to be adapted to the specific client.

Serious Health Issues in the Therapist

I know of several situations in which therapists were seriously compromised, even visibly dying, yet told their anxious patients that there was nothing to worry about (cf. Robbins, 2020). This evasion does immense harm, especially when the clinician "suddenly" dies. The patient then needs to process feelings about the loss, but the one person who understands its magnitude is gone, and people without experience in psychoanalytic treatment rarely understand grief over a loss of this kind. When I am consulted by colleagues with a terminal diagnosis, I remind them that therapy depends on honesty, and that therapists must face the painful burden of addressing their mortality realistically. We need to frankly inform our clients and give them some choice about whether to continue in treatment or to make a termination plan.

My friend Sandra Bem suffered from early Alzheimer's disease. After being diagnosed, she found that despite her memory lapses, many of her psychotherapy clients wanted to go on working with her. In the clinical moment, she was still functional. In response, she had them sign a statement saying that they understood that she was cognitively impaired and were opting nevertheless to continue in treatment. When she began to feel that her mental decline interfered with her being a good-enough therapist, whatever her clients believed, she set an imminent date to retire.

It is increasingly accepted in psychoanalytic circles that analysts should not dissemble, under the pretext of efforts to be "neutral" or "abstinent," about medical realities that might interrupt or end treatment. Barbara Pizer's (1997) writing about her experience sharing a breast cancer diagnosis was pivotal in this shift. As in many areas, conventional nondisclosure norms, originally adopted to open up the analytic process by allowing freer associations and greater access to fantasy, can instead close those processes down when the patient suspects that a potentially treatment-interfering condition is being hidden. Beginning supervisees may not know about the current consensus that the analyst's serious illness may override ordinary conventions of therapeutic discourse, and clinicians at any level of experience may need considerable supervisory support in dealing with all the feelings that painful disclosures set in motion.

ETHICAL DILEMMAS INVOLVING THE PATIENT'S BEST INTEREST

Let me start with two examples of clinical situations that raised compelling ethical concerns. The first arose recently for one of my consultees. It is more dramatic than the daily ethical issues that clinicians face, but in its nature, it is a not an uncommon kind of quandary. The second was a less consequential but still troublesome clinical problem that I once had to deal with, for which consultation proved helpful. Neither situation could have been resolved neatly by reference to ethics codes, and both involved competing moral claims.

1. A Stunning Realization and Its Multiple Potential Consequences

A colleague in South America, who occasionally confers with me about his cases, asked for my assistance in deciding how to handle issues that had arisen in his work with a woman whom he had taken into treatment several months earlier. She had come for relief from recurrent depressions, unalleviated by medication, and for help improving her troubled relationships with men, which she attributed to having been brought up without a father.

My colleague had felt an immediate sense of affection toward this client. She was poised and attractive, and in their initial session, the thought had passed through his mind that she resembled a beloved old friend who lived far away, whom he hadn't seen in years. The patient connected her depression with several experiences with male teachers, bosses, and lovers in which she had found herself eventually feeling neglected, misunderstood, and/or rejected. Her current intimate relationship with a man felt fragile to her. At the time the therapist called me, he and the patient had been meeting twice weekly, and their working alliance seemed solid.

This woman, now a professor of literature, had been raised in dire economic circumstances. In her family of origin there had been no father or paternal figure; her mother had told her that she was the product of a one-night stand, and that she had no idea where her father was now. My colleague noted to himself that this history shed valuable light on his client's expectation of rejection, depressive self-hatred, and recurrent problems with men. The therapy was going well, and the clinician was beginning to address the patient's transferential fears that he did not care about her and would eventually reject her.

In their session preceding his call to me, she had spoken for the first time of a brief period after college when she had been an academic intern in another country. Her field of study was highly specialized, even esoteric. She had thought there would be no money for the internship and was surprised when her mother somehow came up with funds. A vivid memory suddenly invaded my colleague's mind: His old friend, the one the client resembled, had long ago confided, after several drinks, that he had once cheated on his wife, with the result that he was the biological father of an adult daughter who lived near the city where my consultee now practices. He stated that the girl's mother knew where he was but had contacted him only once, to ask him to pay for their daughter's internship in the obscure academic area and distant country my colleague's patient had mentioned. In return for this financial support, the mother had allowed him to view the young woman from a distance and had pointed out her resemblance to him. The age, field of study, and current residence of my supervisee's patient all dovetailed exactly with his old friend's story.

Parenthetically, such uncanny coincidences are less rare than one might think. More ordinary dilemmas of a similar nature are not uncommon; intrusions on treatment by information coming from outside the office cause clinical headaches with which therapists are painfully familiar. Most of us have been in the uncomfortable situation of having become privy to critical facts about a client that the client does not have. This can happen even when we are being scrupulous about boundaries. For example, we are working with a person who turns out to know someone else in our caseload, who mentions some pertinent data about which both we and the other client had been ignorant. Or we learn through a personal grapevine that a patient's partner is having an unsuspected affair.

My supervisee knew with almost complete certainty who his patient's abandoning father was. What should he do? Should he tell her? Supporting that option is the fact that secrets tend to undermine the free inquiry that is critical to the therapy process. If I am innocent of knowledge that my patient's husband is cheating, and I hear from her about peculiar changes in his behavior, I might ask, "Have you ever considered the possibility that he is having an affair?" With insider knowledge, however, this question is no longer innocently exploratory. I would hence be unlikely to ask it. The unbidden knowledge inhibits my freedom to raise possibilities. It is extremely burdensome to know something important that a patient does not know, and in this situation, one inevitably feels vaguely dishonest with the client.

My South American colleague was facing a challenging moral dilemma. He had a long-standing obligation to his friend, to whom he had pledged never to reveal his secret. But he had a pressing professional commitment to the ultimate welfare of his client. It might be argued that one's duties to a patient override a promise made long ago to a friend. But the therapist had no way of weighing the potential negative consequences of betraying his friend's confidence against the potential negative effects on his patient (and, for that matter, on her mother and her mother's family) if he should opt to tell her what he knew about her probable paternity.

The Hippocratic principle "First, do no harm" seemed to militate against revealing what he knew. And yet what if, at some future point, the client were to talk with the therapist about an intention to find out who her father is? What if she wanted to search for him and meet with him? How could the therapist support such a plan in good faith? Absent the connection to his friend, he might have taken the general psychoanalytic position that knowledge, however painful, is preferable to ignorance. With what he knew, however, he had a certain emotional stake in her ignorance that could compromise his usual professional stance.

What if the patient were eventually to discover her father's identity and learn from him that her therapist had been his friend and confidante? Would she be appalled that the therapist had never revealed this stunning information? Would she feel as betrayed by my colleague as she might already feel by her father for his having left her and by her mother for having lied to her about not knowing his whereabouts? Would such a revelation undo many years of devoted therapy? Such disasters have been known to happen, and most of us would put a high priority on preventing them. Real ethical dilemmas are often messy in these ways.

Given that we could not predict the consequences of disclosure, the therapist and I decided he should not say anything. Unlike a decision to tell the secret, which could never be undone, this position could be changed in the future. We rationalized that because even though it was 99% probable that his friend was his patient's father, he could not ignore the 1% possibility to the contrary. It remains to be seen how his forthcoming work with this woman will be affected by his private knowledge, but at least he knows I am available to share the burden of future decisions that may arise about this patient's best interests.

An interesting feature of this quandary is its conflict between personal and professional moral claims: The destruction of a valued friendship in the name of clinical ethics is certainly not morally neutral, but it sometimes happens when therapists see no alternative to putting the client's welfare above a personal relationship. In the example that follows, a more trivial version of this kind of conflict, I suffered a minor degree of marital strain because of a clinical situation.

2. A Problematic Enactment

Many years ago, I was contacted for treatment by a man who lived in my neighborhood, from which I ordinarily did not take patients (maintaining a professional appearance and proper discipline in the office is demanding enough; having to maintain them everywhere else because I might run into a patient is a burden I prefer to avoid). But this man specifically wanted to talk to a psychoanalyst, and there were few analytically trained therapists within easy commuting distance. And what he wanted to work on was unresolved grief about the death of his mother from cancer when he was a boy, something I felt I could help him with because of the loss of my own mother to cancer around the same age. We carefully compared our social networks, decided there was no overlap that would interfere with my being his therapist, and made a contract to work together. I have his permission to include the following situation in this book.

In the second year of his therapy, my patient decided to run for public office. The head of his local political party happened to be my former husband, Carey (now deceased), who began talking to me about this promising new candidate. Confidentiality precluded my saying anything, but I began to feel deceptive when the campaign came up in household conversations, for example, when I had to invent excuses to reject my husband's suggestion that we invite the candidate to dinner. My patient was enjoying and learning from his connection with my husband, and the patient and I were talking about what it was bringing up for him to be working with his therapist's spouse. I began feeling that it was unfair that my husband was ignorant of the situation, and I was dissimulating at home to a degree that made me uncomfortable.

I consulted a colleague, who suggested that I ask the patient to tell Carey in confidence that he was seeing me in treatment. He reminded me that confidentiality belongs to the patient, who has the right to decide to waive it. Because I, in contrast, have the right to breach confidentiality only in the direst circumstances, I had not thought of any possibility involving disclosure. I followed my colleague's advice and, fortunately, my patient was willing to comply with my request. The arrangement worked out fairly well, although the revelation made my husband irritable and prickly for a while, both at me for my uncharacteristic prevarications and at his political protégé for what he saw as his provocative secrecy. Fortunately, he himself had been in psychoanalysis and could appreciate both the patient's situation and my own professional dilemma, and so his irritation soon dissipated.

If my client had refused to tell my spouse about his clinical relationship with me, I wonder how I would have handled the situation. If his political relationship with my husband had involved consequences severe enough to make it impossible for me to do my job effectively, I could have legitimately made our continuing work together conditional on his speaking to him. Later in this chapter, I focus on ethical and practical claims that therapists are entitled to make on their own behalf to protect their functioning in their clinical role. But because the situation was only awkward, not significantly injurious, I would likely have soldiered on, trying to analyze the enactment with the patient and hoping that he would begin to feel self-conscious enough to come clean eventually to his political mentor about his connection to his wife.

Some colleagues may have taken the position that once my client decided to be a candidate for public office and knew that his decision would involve a relationship with my husband, we should have stopped working together clinically. One could argue that I should have framed his situation as a choice between his political ambitions and his treatment, emphasizing that he could run for office after his therapy ended. But his decision to seek public office was part of his therapeutic improvement, he did not have the option to do so outside our mutual locality, and my husband was realistically the proper advisor for his political aims.

Forcing a choice between therapy and politics would have felt to me punitive, beyond my scope of authority in his life, and undermining of his progress. Treatment was not at a natural end point, and if he were to choose to terminate in favor of his political aims, he would have suffered the replication of an early loss that had greatly influenced his psychological problems. (Also, I suspect that my inclinations reflected my feeling that my client would do a great job in the office he was pursuing. This sense was not relevant to the ethical evaluation, and its effects were mostly unconscious, but I mention that fact in the interest of full disclosure. Incidentally, he was elected and, from my perspective, governed well—outcomes that I would like to think may have been at least slightly influenced by his work with me.)

Both of these vignettes speak to the importance of supervision and consultation, even for experienced therapists. Both required more than one mind to consider the diverse options and their possible ramifications. Neither dilemma has an obvious, morally unambiguous resolution without any potential downside. But despite their complexities, these instances of ethical challenge are easier than those that involve the additional supervisory functions of gatekeeping and protection of the public. The main people affected by the therapist's decision in the prior examples are the therapist, the patient, and some individuals in intimate relationships with them. Let me turn to an instance in which the boundary between treatment and social consequences is more problematic.

ETHICAL DILEMMAS INVOLVING
THE COMMUNITY'S BEST INTERESTS

Requests for the Therapist's Practical Help or Advocacy

I was recently asked by a relatively inexperienced supervisee how he should respond to a patient's request that he write a letter supporting her application for disability status. She wanted him to say that she had a severe personality disorder (she did meet DSM criteria for such a diagnosis) and was too depressed to pursue employment. If she were able to secure an official classification as disabled, she would have a guaranteed income from the government. The therapist had worked hard to convince this distrusting, sullen client that he was a sympathetic, supportive, potentially helpful listener. He found himself inclined to say yes, but he thought he should talk to me about it before assenting. He noted in passing that he was not looking forward to crafting such a letter.

The patient was in her early 20s, living with her family of origin after having graduated from college with average grades. She seemed to be suffering a "failure to launch": She was sleeping late, feeling apathetic, and spending most of her time in Internet chat rooms. Although she was clearly depressed, she had been unresponsive to prescribed antidepressant medications. She took a notably passive stance in treatment, implying that any therapist who cared about her would want to make her life easier by endorsing her appropriateness for ongoing fiscal support.

My supervisee was conscientiously observant of the American Psychological Association's (2017) ethical principles of beneficence, fidelity/responsibility, integrity, justice, and respect for people's rights and dignity. At first glance, it appeared to him that *beneficence* would lie in granting his patient's request: His doing so would demonstrate his appreciation of her depressed state and his empathy for her feeling of hopelessness, messages he thought would strengthen the therapeutic alliance. But our conversation about the situation exposed the fact that he did not really regard this young woman as incapable of working. To say in a letter that he viewed her as permanently disabled would therefore not be entirely true and would violate the foundational ethical principle of *integrity*. It would set a less-than-honest example for the patient, who tended to prevaricate rather than relating straightforwardly to others.

As we talked, the supervisee disclosed his long-standing personal difficulty in disappointing others, a tendency he attributed to having been raised by parents who had undermined his own efforts at individuation. He wondered whether he might be rationalizing doing what was easy instead of what was therapeutic. Might beneficence actually lie in telling the patient, frankly but tactfully, that despite the fact that she was in a depressed state, he did not see her as disabled? He dreaded the outrage that would almost certainly follow his declining to do her bidding, and he knew from past experience that she would equate his saying no with his disgustedly rejecting her as a person.

In this instance, the supervisee's countertransference provided valuable data about whether complying with the client's demand was truly an ethical position. In our conversation, he became aware that the request had made him feel uneasy and a bit "slimy." He was able to take that reaction seriously, wonder about what it was telling him, and get in touch with his suspicion that he was being asked to be an enabler of this woman's psychopathology. On examination, the patient's wishes seemed to involve far more than an uncomplicated favor that any caring professional should readily grant.

This young woman had started treatment acknowledging ingrained tendencies toward regressive, avoidant reactions to life's challenges. She and the therapist had agreed that a goal of therapy should be increasing her sense of agency. He and I wondered together whether her entreaty contained what control-mastery theorists construe as an unconscious test (Silberschatz, 2005), and if so, what the nature of the test was. On the surface, the test seemed to be "Do you care enough about me to write a letter on my behalf?" This conceptualization amounted to a "transference test" (Weiss, 1993), in which the patient would be essentially saying, "Are you going to fail the test by invalidating me the way my mother always did, or are you going to pass it by offering nonjudgmental acceptance?"). But that explanation did not feel right or complete, because both therapist and patient had agreed that therapy would involve a developmental process in which the client would reverse her retreat from adulthood and gradually attain more autonomous functioning.

At a deeper level, we thought the test might be something like: "Will you demonstrate that under pressure you can be more self-advocating and firm than I have ever been able to be? Will you fail, by doing the easy thing [saying yes], or will you pass the test, by taking a harder position, one that risks my rage but views me with respect, as someone capable of eventually being a contributing member of the human community?" This possibility felt more resonant to my supervisee. He began to suspect that the test was mainly of another type, a "passive-into-active transformation" (Weiss, 1993), in which patients pose a dilemma typical of their formative years and see whether the therapist can do something better with it than they were able to do growing up. This woman had often complained that she could never object to something that her parents pushed her to do, and the therapist had been feeling, in what Racker (1968) would call a concordant countertransference, that he could not object to his client's demand.

The therapist began to realize that even though she would not immediately experience a rejection of her request as embodying the ethical tenet of *respect for the patient's dignity,* that principle required him to treat her as a potentially fully functioning adult. (In *Psychoanalytic Psychotherapy* [McWilliams, 2004], I discuss a similar situation in which my patient "Donna" slowly came to understand my saying no as *respect.*) My supervisee's client had learned to influence other people's behavior by reacting to reasonable limits with tantrums, and most authorities, including those in her family of origin, tended to cave in to her demands, because it was easier than setting boundaries that would require her to make more mature adaptations to life's challenges.

The therapist and I also looked at the question of whether writing a letter seeking disability status would amount to his being in an ethically problematic dual role, in this case, being both an advocate and a therapist. Sometimes clinicians need to advocate for a patient. When that is true, such support can be integrated readily with one's clinical role and does not feel "dual." For example, with the client's permission, a therapist might intervene with an insurance company to ensure authorization of sufficient sessions, or with a child's parent or teacher with suggestions of ways to help, or with a physician to share observations of the patient's symptoms. In other situations, especially in some institutional settings, therapists are required to make specific reports, a condition of the treatment that should be acknowledged as part of the frame from the outset. In that case, there is no clinical decision to make.

But in many instances, being a therapist and acting as an advocate are at odds with each other, are not in the best interest of the patient, and do constitute the kind of dual role that ethics codes rightly discourage or prohibit. A clinician's joining a patient's side in a legal battle, for example, can severely compromise treatment, even when the therapist is convinced of the righteousness of the client's position. Supervisors and consultants often need to teach even experienced clinicians that advocacy creates special complications for psychodynamic work. The "basic rule" of analytic treatment asks the client to say everything. If a patient were to feel that her therapist might pursue applying for disability status or testify in court on her behalf, she would be tempted, consciously and unconsciously, to skew her communications toward thoughts and feelings that support this aim, exiling all other aspects of her subjective world to a desert island at which no rescue boats ever arrive. In Chapter 2, I noted the foolhardiness of the requirement in the early analytic institutes that candidates' personal analysts report on their suitability for progressing through levels of training and eventual graduation. This issue is comparable.

The therapist and I concluded that the ethical position here (and, happily, the therapeutic one) would be to refuse the patient's request. We then talked about how best to give her the disappointing news while maintaining empathic attunement to her conscious state of mind. For example, he might tell the patient, "I have complete sympathy with your wish to get this kind of support, but my problem with complying is that I can't honestly say that you are permanently unable to work. Once you and I work through your depression and your anxieties about putting yourself forward in the world, I would want you to feel the self-esteem involved in earning your own way. I know you are despairing enough right now not to be able to see such a future, but I do."

Then we talked about how one can live through the rage of a vengeful patient, which was predictable in this case. This might include such options as (1) just sucking it up and surviving the affect storms, (2) noting that it is painful to be seen as such a sadistic tormenter, and/or (3) commenting on the either–or polarities in which the patient seems stuck. We discussed how the therapist might eventually note this either–or split and raise the question of whether the client could imagine him as having any possible motive other than these binary options. He could say, for example, "You seem to be convinced that there are only two possibilities: Either I care about you enough to do this, or I hate you. Can you imagine my having any other motive?"

Toward the end of this long supervisory conversation, I reminisced about times when a frustrated patient excoriated me for weeks or months, but later told me that my saying no to some request had exemplified a firm, self-possessed stance that the patient was later able to call to mind and inhabit when faced with unreasonable demands or personal mistreatment. I associated to one woman whose impassioned request for a hug I rejected. She was outraged for weeks, but she later told me that her identification with my boundaries had subsequently enabled her to stand up to her abusive husband. I hoped that a vision of an eventual good outcome for a clinical position that was hard for this man to take would increase his self-assurance in setting what we had agreed was a therapeutic limit.

Michael Garrett (2019), who because of his work with more disturbed patients in a hospital setting receives many such requests, tells me that his first concern is to change the situation from one in which patients passively expect him to do something for the them into one in which agency lies within the patient. With a man who asks for a disability letter, he will first ask how he has thought through what he needs. How would he describe his "disability," and what does it disable him from doing? Some hospital patients will deny any psychiatric diagnosis, in which case that denial is what he and the patient will first discuss; disability is off the table until that issue is resolved. In other words, it is food for therapeutic thought if the patient is seeking disability on the basis of a diagnosis that the patient does not accept.

With patients who can make a case that they have a disability, he asks about their remediation plan. His hospital is in New York, where disability status is reviewed at regular intervals by government employees. Patients are responsible for having a plan to remediate their problem and reporting about that plan regularly (he also discusses creating a plan with patients who have none). With patients who have not been complying with the details of a prior plan (remediation plans typically stipulate that the patient come regularly to appointments and take prescribed medications), he will start a conversation about why they are not holding up their part of the compact that they have made with the state.

In cases in which sending a letter is legitimate, such as instances in which the patient is severely psychiatrically disabled and participating conscientiously in a remediation plan, he will write a letter but insist that the patient read it carefully before he sends it. This practice has evolved from experiences in which psychotic patients do not recognize themselves, become upset, and speak about suing for false representation. His having them approve the letter complies with HIPAA regulations about patients' right to know and, in addition, prevents reactions such as "You screwed me!" or "Why didn't you include such-and-such?" And while they are reviewing the letter with him, important clinical material may emerge.

The previous example concerns the supervisor's responsibility to the community when clients seek benefits that their fellow citizens support with taxes. More serious situations involving therapists' duties to

124PSYCHOANALYTIC SUPERVISION

the larger society are increasingly common in the United States and other Western countries. In recent decades, a growing body of legislation requires clinicians to play a role in preventing suicide, homicide, and child abuse. My students increasingly struggle with questions of when and how to contact public authorities, especially when children may be in danger. Seasoned therapists are additionally burdened by experiences of inadequacies in the social service agencies they report to; they know that the likeliest outcome of their calling the authorities will be the destruction of the therapeutic alliance. Everyone in our field struggles with these situations, and no supervisor can be an expert on all the possibilities.

Risk Management for Therapists and Supervisors

In addition to examining problems in individual and/or group consultation, the best direction that supervisors can give to therapists wrestling with such issues includes advising them to seek out ethics specialists in their professional organizations or malpractice insurance agencies. These services are usually free. When legal questions are involved, or when a state board has received a complaint from a disgruntled patient about a clinician, supervisors should urge the therapist to pay for consultation with an attorney trained in mental health law. Preferably, it should be someone who also has some experience with (and ideally a credential in) psychotherapy. Such experts are rare and immensely valuable; mentors should caution supervisees that lawyers without a feel for clinical work tend to move quickly toward risk management for the therapist without a consideration of what will benefit the patient and the possibilities of maintaining the therapeutic alliance.

It interests me how seldom therapists think spontaneously about getting legal help when they struggle with the interface between treatment and other social claims. Less experienced therapists may feel that having been educated about pertinent laws and regulations, they should know by now what to do; they may feel that asking for this help makes them look inadequate. Experienced therapists tend not to think of reaching out to legal experts because they are used to solving their problems within the clinical and counseling communities. It can be enormously relieving to anyone grappling with responsibilities beyond the consulting room to realize that there are other available professionals who have relevant and valuable expertise.

On the topic of relationships with attorneys, let me add that when they are contacted by lawyers or courts early in their careers, clinicians tend to become very anxious and often need help from more seasoned therapists and experts in mental health law. When asked for records, in the service of confidentiality, they should submit the minimum data their state allows. Newer therapists are not yet aware that lawyers may ask for more information than they are entitled to, hoping that clinicians are ignorant of legal limitations. When an attorney requests a clinician's testimony in a conflict such as a divorce, even when patients want to waive confidentiality so that the therapist can speak on their behalf, mentors should emphasize that there is no such thing as a partial waiver of confidentiality. A clinician wiling to testify that a client was bullied by her husband, for example, would have to admit in court that she also talked in therapy about her own infidelities.

Supervisors can often help clinicians with proper documentation so that they are at minimal risk when legal matters complicate their role. Courts tend to understand the limitations of clinical understanding and influence. Therapists are allowed to be wrong, but they are required to be thoughtful. They need to understand community standards for record-keeping, to document their thoughtfulness about whatever positions they have taken with the patient, to note in the record who is responsible for what aspect of the person's treatment, and to document consultations with experienced colleagues when they fear that a patient will act in ways that provoke legal consequences. Thus, supervisees can be told that a good way to minimize risk is to write clinical notes in the following form: "In addressing the clinical dilemma, I considered two possibilities. On the one hand . . . ; On the other hand . . . ; After thoroughly considering both options and consulting with a colleague, I made the decision to do X."

Evaluation of Trainees

When supervisees are not yet credentialed for independent practice, or when they are in postgraduate institute training, the supervisor's role typically includes periodic formal evaluation of their progress. (It also often includes writing letters of recommendation, to which similar considerations apply.) Mentors struggle to find the right balance between supporting positive elements and criticizing negative elements of the supervisee's work. It can be tempting, especially with students whose self-esteem seems fragile, to give generally complimentary reviews, or to put positive material in the record and privately and informally note a few reservations to the authorities in their programs.

A supervisor's avoidance of fully honest criticism puts program authorities in a difficult position. It patronizes the supervisee as well.

Because students of analytic therapies have to get used to speaking frankly, albeit tactfully, to vulnerable patients, their supervisors' evasion of doing so with them deprives them of models of straight talk. As Otto Kernberg (2010) observes, "Some supervisors find it difficult to combine teaching within a collegial atmosphere while critically evaluating the candidate, and yet that is the essential task of supervisors" (p. 604).

Although it is not always legally required, I feel strongly that supervisory evaluations should be shared with trainees before they are officially submitted. This practice gives mentors practice in framing constructive criticism tactfully (a useful skill throughout one's career). It gives students time to deal with their feelings about the supervisor's comments, to become conscious of mixed or negative reactions, and to discuss differences of opinion. If a student persuades the supervisor to rethink the report, it can be revised accordingly; when a disagreement cannot be resolved, the supervisee can put a personal statement in the file—a kind of "minority report" on the supervisory experience.

At the end of any prescribed period of supervision, the trainee should also be expected to evaluate the supervisor, much as college students are asked to evaluate their professors at the end of each course. Despite the fact that any good mentor will have periodically invited the mentee's opinion about how the supervision is working out and what the supervisee sees as the supervisor's respective strengths and weaknesses, most students will withhold the "whole truth" from such conversations. Because of the potentially devastating effects on their career of a negative review from a supervisor, it is not reasonable to expect supervisees to be completely candid, especially if one of their complaints is that the supervisor seems too narcissistic to tolerate differences of opinion.

But they should be able to tell some responsible person in their training program about their misgivings and, in this case, given the influence a disgruntled supervisor may have on a student's professional life, they should expect the details of their complaints to be kept private. Directors of training programs are duty bound not only to protect the public from destructive clinicians, but also to protect their candidates from potentially destructive supervisors. In supervision groups of more than four, in which the authors of evaluations are anonymous, faculty supervisors can learn a lot from reading the participants' critiques of their supervision. In one-on-one settings, in contrast, the supervised therapist tends to be identifiable and thus vulnerable to retaliation. Thoughtful program directors appreciate these realities and find ways of quietly not assigning students to supervisors who have been given more than one significantly negative review.

Gatekeeping

Because they tend to be generous people who enjoy the gratifications of supervisees' appreciation, most mentors probably view it as the realization of their worst nightmares when they suspect that a supervisee is a potential danger to clients or the public. Thankfully, in my experience this is rare. But I recall two memorable times, during my 40 years of teaching in a clinical psychology graduate program, when the faculty ultimately had to face this reality. In both cases it stressed us out to do so; we hated to give up on a student, and we faced splits and misunderstandings among ourselves that made reaching a decision difficult.

The first situation involved a young heterosexual male student who experienced most of his female patients (notably the attractive ones) as having powerful erotic transferences to him. He encouraged them, in what sounded to his peers and teachers like a seductive tone, to talk about their sexual experiences and fantasies, especially as they might involve him. All his supervisors reported that they found his accounts of clinical interactions a little creepy. He had no awareness of the possibility that he was misperceiving many of these clients in an exploitive way, in the service of his own vanity and voyeurism.

When a supervisor questioned the likelihood that every nice-looking woman he treated was in fact immediately filled with sexual desire for him, he suggested that the supervisor was motivated by envy of his youth and attractiveness—and maybe hadn't read enough Freud. He tried to make alliances with the psychoanalytically oriented members of the faculty, stoking their competition with professors of other orientations, and protesting that sexual transference is a time-honored clinical phenomenon that "we" appreciate and "they" do not. (There is some truth in this claim, but erotic transferences are certainly not inevitable or universal, and they rarely arise in the first few sessions. When they do, they tend to signify not so much desire as an effort to exert power, based on experiences in which people of the therapist's gender dominated the client.)

In the case of this student, after trying to get through to him for a couple of years, we learned from staff members at one of his externships that he had behaved dishonestly in ways that more concretely attested to his unsuitability to be a therapist. After keeping a paper trail that would protect our program from losing a lawsuit if this man were to initiate one, we dismissed him from training. Interestingly, instead of being worried about what this action might mean for their own survival in the program, his fellow students reported a sense of relief. As is generally true, they could spot a manipulator long before those of us in authority, whom he was good at deceiving, figured it out.

The other case involved a woman student who seemed deaf to emotion and nuance. She was brilliant, had an extraordinary academic record, and cared deeply about mental health issues. But she could not seem to establish a warm relationship with clients. Her patients complained that she came across as uninterested in everything about them except the conformity of their symptoms to DSM categories. Almost all of them left treatment after one or two sessions. Unlike the previous student, this woman was aware of her interpersonal limitations; she suggested she might be "on the [autism] spectrum" and thus not capable of reading certain interpersonal cues. Although she remained in our program and graduated from it, we were able to help her find a path to doing high-level research in psychopathology instead of pursuing licensure for clinical work.

There are many other situations in which supervisors address ethical matters at the boundary between the clinic and the culture in which it exists. Ethical issues that occur in analytic institutes, a territory I explore in the next chapter, are particularly thorny. I have not included here any thoughts about the supervision one might do at the behest of a regulatory board, when a colleague has been required to be in supervision for a period of time because of what the board deems questionable ethical judgment. I have no experience with that kind of work and would only be guessing about its particular challenges.

ETHICAL DILEMMAS INVOLVING
THE THERAPIST'S BEST INTERESTS

Therapists have legitimate moral and practical claims to conditions of labor that make it possible for them to do their job. It is hardly controversial that those of us treating patients with a history of violence should see them in an office with a nearby security guard or in an agency with an established protocol for responding immediately to a patient's threat to do physical harm. The priority of ensuring the therapist's safety and comfort is clear in such situations. Nonviolent clients can also act, however, in ways that call for certain protections. They may badger patients in the waiting room, or arrive at sessions intoxicated, or "friend" one's child on Facebook to learn intimate family details. The client of one of my colleagues joined her therapist's swimming club so that she could watch her change into her bathing suit. As I noted in Chapter 1, I find that training programs do not always prepare beginning therapists well for setting limits, and I have been impressed with the critical role of supervisors in helping new clinicians do so.

In this chapter, I emphasize limit setting not so much for its value in supporting the therapy process as for its serving the ethical priority of safeguarding the clinician's right to be treated fairly and with basic consideration. Supervisors and consultants sometimes have to challenge unstated but powerful attitudes in therapists that it is only the patient who is entitled to respectful treatment. It often does not occur to supervisees, who spend so much effort trying to take the perspective of the other, that they have a legitimate claim to personal comfort and safety in doing their jobs. Instead, they may implicitly believe they should tolerate any behavior from a patient, especially if they have a sympathetic understanding of its causes.

In their first meetings with clients, it is not generally hard for therapists, even beginners, to specify the "ground rules" that govern the treatment and support the therapist's capacity to work. These differ from one clinician and setting to another; for example, many therapists forbid smoking in their offices, and some ask clients to take off their shoes. But what does become difficult is dealing with impingements that arise during the course of the work. For example, a woman in treatment with one of my colleagues cultivated a friendship with the therapist's adolescent daughter by joining an Alcoholics Anonymous group that she had learned the young woman attended. Chatting her up without mentioning her relationship to her father, she extracted numerous details about his family and began talking excitedly about them in their sessions.

The therapist felt invaded but helpless: He believed he could not interfere with the client's autonomy and pursuit of sobriety. But he was distracted by thoughts of the patient gossiping about his private family issues and enraged by her exploitation of his child. He told a consultant that her behavior was not fair to his daughter, but interestingly, he did not frame the situation as an addressable violation of his own boundaries. The consultant urged him to tell his patient that if she wanted to stay in therapy with him, she would have to attend a different AA meeting. This way of approaching the situation felt like a revelation to him.

When he took this position with the patient, she accused him of being controlling and authoritarian. She mobilized indignant excuses for her behavior, contending that this was the only AA meeting she could conveniently attend and predicting that his daughter would be hurt by her abrupt disappearance. The clinician stated that his comfort mattered as well, that he had a right to privacy, and that if he were to function effectively as her therapist, he had to make her treatment conditional on her not pursuing relationships with members of his family. He went on to say that if he were in a state of resentment about her using his family members to learn intimate details of his life, he could not feel the uncomplicated investment in her welfare that was necessary for their work to succeed. She was angry, but the working through of that anger eventually moved the treatment forward. Later, she grudgingly noted her respect for his ability to defend himself against another person's intrusion, something she had been unable to do growing up. In this case, as is frequently true, what was good for the therapist was also good for the patient.

In a less mutually beneficial instance, I recall a situation in which the therapist made a comparable rule that the patient refused to obey. The clinician terminated the treatment, assisted by advice from a psychologist-attorney who helped her protect herself against future complaints or lawsuits that the client, who had a background of vengeful payback to anyone who thwarted her, might initiate. Therapists often have a deep, multiply-determined need to help every person who walks into their offices, even those who, for psychological and other reasons that a clinician may not be powerful enough to contravene, cannot stop trying to destroy the treatment and/or the therapist. Supervisees need to be told that they are justified in sometimes concluding that a therapeutic relationship is not working. They can be reminded of the ethical principle that we should not continue to take patients' money when we see no evidence of therapeutic change, and they can cite this principle with clients.

During the height of the COVID-19 pandemic in 2020, one of my younger supervisees was working with a man who defiantly announced his refusal to wear a face mask, including when he visited his elderly grandparents. He regarded the pandemic as a fantasy of left-wing media, and he saw no problem with his behavior. The therapist, however, viewed it as dangerous to himself and others and found herself recurrently distracted by her concerns. Finally, she took her feelings to her consultation group, whose members observed that her apprehensions about his behavior were interfering with her capacity to do her job. They told her she had the right to differ with him about wearing masks and to insist that if he were to continue working with her, he would have to agree to cover his face when he went out, because her own comfort in her role required her to insist on his behaving less destructively according to her definition of destructiveness. (I remember one member comparing this intervention to insisting with a pedophile that, even though he saw his behavior as motivated by love and therefore by definition not harmful, treatment would be predicated on his agreement to stop molesting children.)

The clinician felt great relief—and no small amount of surprise—that she could legitimately make such a rule. She told the patient that she respected his right to his own beliefs, but *her* belief that he was imperiling himself and others made her feel she was enabling the spread of the virus if she did not insist on his following the advice of scientists. These worries were occupying mental space that she wanted back. If he wished to work with her, he would have to respect her sensibilities even though he disagreed. He grudgingly consented. Later he confessed that her directive had been advantageous. He had framed his refusal to cover his face in terms of "masculine strength," and he was not going to "look weak" by wearing a mask voluntarily. But, like a teenager who is secretly grateful for a parent's curfew, after she confronted him, he could tell others that his snowflake of a doctor was making him do it and he had to humor her.

In this post-Google era, when limits and boundaries are increasingly porous and basic privacy cannot always be assumed, it is particularly important that therapists pay attention to their ground rules for personal safety and comfort. It would be hard to overstate the value of supervisors' insistence that the therapists in their care consider what is the right behavior that they are owed, and not simply what is ethical practice with respect to others. As in most areas, the major influence on the capacity of therapists to practice adequate self-care is the example of supervisors who do so.

EXEMPLIFYING ETHICAL PRACTICE

As with self-care, the most critical way a supervisor can teach high ethical standards generally is adhere to and model them personally. This should probably go without saying, but evidently it cannot be emphasized enough. Surveys of graduate students have found that supervision is often hampered by trainees' perceptions of their mentors as dishonest, as insufficiently attentive to boundaries, and as involved in various forms of unethical conduct (January, Meyerson, Reddy, Docherty, & Klonoff, 2014). The empirical literature on self-disclosure by therapists in training to supervisors reveals that perceived ethical misconduct by supervisors is a primary cause of supervisees' reluctance to share sensitive aspects of their own psychology and behavior in the supervisory relationship (Mehr et al., 2015). As in all things psychological, what one is told is a lot less impactful than what one is shown.

CONCLUDING COMMENTS

This chapter has addressed some questions of morality and ethics for which supervisory input can make a critical difference, particularly to therapists in the early stages of their careers but also to seasoned practitioners seeking consultation on unique dilemmas. I have offered some orienting thoughts about clinical ethics and patients' rights to know pertinent information. Using detailed vignettes, I have explored how to help therapists deal with ethical challenges that arise with patients. I have discussed the supervision of clinicians' responsibilities toward the larger community and the surrounding society, highlighting the common experience of being asked by clients to advocate for them. I have addressed supervisory obligations with respect to evaluation and professional gatekeeping. I have argued that many clinicians need mentorship in the area of applying to themselves the ethical perspectives they typically work so hard to apply to others. Finally, I have emphasized the importance of the supervisor's exemplification of personal and professional integrity.

In the following chapter, I address the special complexities and challenges of supervision in psychoanalytic institutes, where boundary issues can be much more complicated, and the goals of supervisory consultation more subjective and less clearly articulated than in most other educational settings.

Chapter Seven

■ ■ ■ ■

Supervision in Psychoanalytic Institutes

A friend whose prescience I admire recently emailed me about the challenges of being a training analyst in her institute.

> I think there are differences between supervising candidates and supervising clinicians in the community. With candidates, there are lots of institutional dynamics and multiple relationships at play. A supervisee is not a patient, but there are transferences and vulnerabilities and power differences. I often find myself wondering if it is a betrayal of the supervisory relationship to talk to a colleague who knows the supervisee about some challenge I'm having or even some way I am impressed with the supervisee. And yet, the supervisory relationship can be so complex and confusing and the terrain so not well laid out educationally that I feel especially in need of consultation with colleagues I respect. Like most of us, I've had many years of supervision on working with patients but almost none on supervising.

This brief communication captures almost all the issues I address in this chapter:

- Overt and covert institutional pressures influencing supervision

- Group dynamics germane to supervising in psychoanalytic institutes

- Supervisory transferences and countertransferences

- Boundary issues generally and confidentiality issues specifically

- Impacts on supervision of ill-defined evaluation criteria

- Need for research and training on institute supervision

I begin with general observations about the plusses and minuses of supervising candidates in psychoanalytic training and then address areas pertinent to my colleague's comments.

GRATIFICATIONS OF SUPERVISING IN PSYCHOANALYTIC INSTITUTES

The role of supervisor, especially of a "training" or "control" analyst in the postgraduate education of psychoanalysts, is enviable in many ways. Mentoring future analysts is intrinsically rewarding: One can work with highly motivated clinicians already grounded in psychoanalytic theory and practice, who can focus on complex and fine-tuned dynamic processes that may elude beginners. These supervisees are already colleagues, in that they already practice psychotherapy, and they will eventually become coworkers on institute committees and coparticipants at institute events. Deep and lasting friendships between supervisors and their previous supervisees are common. For decades, I remained close to one of my control analysts until his death, and I have remained close to the other analyst to the present day.

Supervision of aspiring psychoanalysts benefits from the fact that they have had their own therapy. Some institutes expect candidates to be in treatment throughout their training; others require a certain (usually high) number of hours of personal analysis. A small number of European institutes make personal treatment voluntary, but foster a culture in which everyone expects candidates to seek it. Immersion in one's own analysis helps therapists to integrate their intellectual knowledge with their emotional experience. And because treatment deepens their self-understanding and self-acceptance, they can empathize with a wider range of issues in their patients, go into their countertransference reactions in greater depth, and feel less painfully exposed when sensitive parts of their own psychologies come to light in consultation.

Candidates at analytic institutes tend to be curious, intellectually sophisticated, more highly motivated for in-depth training, and more broadly educated than the average graduate student studying to be a therapist. They may possess interests and backgrounds in philosophy, theology, the arts, and the humanities and the social sciences generally. They are attracted to complexity and depth. They often have ambitions to write about psychotherapy and have great psychological questions. They seek immersion in communities where ideas matter, where relationship is valued, where the effort to be honest about the darkest aspects of being human is a defining communal value. They respect the wisdom that comes from experience along with the knowledge that comes from scientific investigation. They make impressive personal sacrifices to be as fully educated as possible in their craft. Engagement with them in supervision is both intellectually stimulating and emotionally fulfilling.

CHALLENGES OF SUPERVISING IN PSYCHOANALYTIC INSTITUTES

At the same time, as is evident in my friend's email, supervising institute candidates presents unique challenges. They enter analytic training programs hoping not simply to become more skilled as therapists, but to join a community. In a way, they are trying out the experience of belonging to a certain kind of family, but without the advantage of a birthright. And their adaptation to institute training can be difficult. Candidates who were often the most highly regarded individuals in their prior training programs can feel like beginners again as soon as they situate themselves behind a couch. Despite all their past successes, they are vulnerable to feeling unskilled, naïve, and insufficiently prepared for this new role. This situation is further taxed by the fact that there is virtually no agreement in our field about how to define a competent psychoanalyst. Growth toward that elusive goal happens not by learning a consensual corpus of material but via a series of nurturing relationships, which expand one's self-definition beyond previous identifications (Nagell et al., 2014).

In a psychotherapy relationship, the patient and clinician have a kind of equality. The patient pays the therapist's fee, directly or via a clinic or a third party, and the therapist attends to the patient's psychological needs. As many analysts have noted in one phrase or another, psychotherapy relationships are "mutual but asymmetrical" (Aron, 1991), in that the two participants have a kind of moral equality in the relationship despite their differences in perceived power. The same cannot be said for institute supervision. Because of the evaluative role of supervisors, candidates cannot be expected to be as self-disclosing as they ask patients to be, and they are keenly aware of this reality (Cabaniss et al., 2003; Casement, 2005), a problem I say more about shortly.

Candidates in institutes are mature adults—often unusually mature adults—but because they are in personal psychoanalyses that may be activating their earliest and most affectively saturated self-states (see Yerushalmi, 2014), they not infrequently become caught up in enactments of some fairly primitive dynamics on the stage of the institute itself. For example, they may be experiencing and/or evoking splits between supervisors, between their analyst and a supervisor, between their analyst or supervisor and institute authorities, or among their candidate peers. They may displace onto their supervisor some conflictual or defensive responses that their analysis has activated, rather than being able to contain that material within their treatment.

The human tendency to regress in groups has been observed for decades (Bion, 1961; Rice, 1965, 1969) and studied in depth for many years by group and organizational psychologists (e.g., Kets de Vries & Miller, 1984; Menzies, 1960; Schein, 1985). In some institutes, splits originate in paranoiagenic politics specific to that organization (see Kernberg, 1996, 1998). These are inevitably absorbed and elaborated by candidates, whether or not their own personalities or current treatment issues incline them toward primitive projection and splitting (Bruzzone, Casaula, Jimenez, & Jordan, 1985; Kernberg, 2016). In the training programs of the American Psychoanalytic Association, some of these organizational dynamics derive directly from the two-tiered hierarchy of the training analyst system, which creates cultures of hurt feelings, envy, and devaluation (Auchincloss & Michels, 2003; Eisold, 2004; Kernberg, 2016; Kirsner, 2000; Wallerstein, 2010). Supervisors of analytic candidates can thus find themselves in fraught emotional and political situations within their organizations.[1]

---

[1] I am commenting on these hierarchical dynamics as an outsider. Neither the institute where I trained (the National Psychological Association for Psychoanalysis [NPAP]) nor the institute with which I am locally affiliated (the Center for Psychotherapy and Psychoanalysis of New Jersey [CPPNJ]) belongs to the American Psychoanalytic Association (APsaA) or the International Psychoanalytical Association. (As a non-physician, I could not have applied to an institute of the APsaA in 1973 even if I had wanted to, unless I would attest that I wanted the training for academic purposes only, not with an intent to practice.) NPAP viewed its trainees as capable of analyzing and supervising candidates as soon as they graduated. To supervise for CPPNJ, one must be 2 years postgraduation, and to analyze candidates, one must be 5 years out. My institutes have had many fraught controversies and some notable schisms, but they did not arise from a training analyst system (McWilliams, 2016).

Issues of Psychoanalytic Identity

Early in their analytic training, most candidates identify primarily with one theoretical orientation and only gradually assimilate other perspectives into it (see Schafer, 1979, on "becoming an analyst of one persuasion or another"). This process is normative and healthy. It is hard enough to learn one psychoanalytic language, and we all resonate differently to alternative theoretical frameworks and their preferred metaphors. Candidates tend to find, based on their reading and prior experiences in therapy and supervision, that one orientation "speaks to" them more than others do. Out of the universal dynamics that impel human beings to value their own group over others, they then may split between, for example, the good self psychologists and the bad ego psychologists, or the good Lacanians and the bad relationalists, or the good Kleinians and the bad Freudians.

Unfortunately, any smoldering rivalries between senior analysts in an institute can be ignited by these normal processes of identifying with a chosen approach and devaluing other theoretical orientations. The much-lamented tendency for analytic training programs to suffer rifts that then spawn competing institutes may arise at least partly from such dynamics. I suspect that schismatic processes also derive from the fact that in a personal analysis, competitive sibling transferences arise much less frequently than parental transferences and so are less likely to have been worked through in the analyses of candidates (or supervisors). Hence, they may be enacted in groups and systems, which more naturally evoke brother–sister dynamics (see Edwards, 2011).

An additional problem related to identity concerns the freestanding nature of psychoanalytic institutes, a status that reduces their accountability to outside influences. Like all organizations, they tend to self-replicate and to resist change. Unlike universities, for example, which feel external political pressures to continue adapting to social and political developments and to extend themselves to previously underserved groups, analytic institutes have to depend mostly on the persuasiveness of their existing members to do so (for a good example of such persuasiveness, see Holmes, 2016). Cabaniss and colleagues (2001) found that supervisees often choose not to talk to their supervisors about issues of prejudice, marginality, and cultural diversity. I have heard many anecdotes from candidates about feeling patronized when they have been brave enough to tell them (see also Hart, Dunn, & Jones, 2020). The following reminiscence came from a South Asian analyst friend:

I learned slowly to "just" focus on the intrapsychic and genetic origins of what was going on with my Indian patients because if I focused on issues of prejudice, privilege, and power relations, I felt I was making my supervisors, who were all white, uncomfortable. One supervisor even made a pejorative comment about "fresh-off-the-boat, uneducated Bangladeshis," while reassuring me, "Of course, you're in a different league."

It is critical that we help our mentees integrate a psychoanalytic identity into their other self-states, rather than adopt a psychoanalytic identity at the expense of those identifications.

Problematic Consequences of Idealization and Devaluation

As Kohut (1971, 1977) taught us, idealization and deidealization are normal features of human development. We revere people whose values and skills we want to emulate. At first, we want to swallow them whole, and then gradually we retain some of their qualities and reject others (cf. Schafer, 1968). In normative development, idealization does not ultimately become defensive grandiosity, and deidealization does not become defensive devaluation; emotional maturity involves a strong sense of what one believes and values, coexisting with a respect for other perspectives and an acknowledgment of one's own limitations. But in the early phases of assimilating new identifications and attachments, which will eventually be incorporated into one's self-definition and self-esteem, idealization and devaluation can be fairly stark and lacking in nuance. Remnants of that primitivity are easy to see in both individual and organizational psychology. When we supervise in analytic institutes, they require constant monitoring in ourselves as well as in our supervisees.

In my own case, becoming a psychoanalyst was something I pursued with all the passion of a zealot, and being a psychoanalyst continues to be central to my own identity. Consequently, I have to be careful not to take personally any attack on psychoanalysis. And when one of my students rejects psychodynamic ideas in favor of other formulations, even though this decision may signal the person's increasing maturity and capacity for self-direction, I cannot help feeling somewhat personally rejected. (Fortunately, the older I get, the less I am wounded by the fact that other people are separate grown-ups.) The vicissitudes of idealization and devaluation, so central to learning at all ages, create ongoing problems for most supervisors, as well as for psychoanalytic institutes as cultures.

For example, any narcissistically infused commitment of the supervisor to a specific psychoanalytic orientation can be reinforced by candidates seeking to venerate a mentor as an icon of one point of view (Arlow, 1972; Balint, 1948; Roustang, 1982). A supervisor's perspective could also be painfully devalued, of course, but students in institutes can typically choose their supervisors, and they generally choose those who are identified with an orientation they find attractive. For supervisors, one possible outcome of being frequently selected and deferred to by candidates who are looking to idealize a paragon of their favored approach is becoming increasingly dogmatic about their own ways of working.

It is a known occupational hazard of being a training analyst, especially one whose practice consists mostly of analytic candidates, that any tendencies one has toward defensive self-inflation thrive on a constant diet of idealization (Arlow, 1972; Eisold, 2004; Kernberg, 2010; Roustang, 1982; Vollmer & Bernardi, 1996). In supervision, when both mentor and mentee see clinical material through only one lens, technique may become inflexible, and different ways of handling therapeutic challenges may be ignored to the potential detriment of both the patient and the supervisee (see, e.g., Lauro et al., 2003).

Patients may be a bad "fit" with a favored model and may need to be understood and influenced from more than one angle of vision. These days, our field is notable for its pluralism (Birkhofer, 2017; Wallerstein, 1992), but this state of affairs can be confusing to beginning analysts, who often seek consistency and idealize those who seem to "know" which approach is best (see Rangell, 1982). Candidates who idealize a supervisor may not want to notice potential differences of opinion between themselves and their mentor, in which case they run the risk of becoming a psychoanalytic clone rather than an integrated, separate professional. In older psychoanalytic language, instead of their ego functions expanding, their superego functions rigidify (Balint, 1948; Hanoch, 2006; Kernberg, 1996). There is no inherent problem with supervisors representing, and identifying closely with, one psychoanalytic orientation; that identity provides definition and clarity to trainees. But we need to take care not to belittle other approaches and thereby leave our supervisees defensively and inflexibly identified (or defensively and inflexibly counteridentified) with our point of view.

Issues involving supervisees' idealization and/or devaluation of their own analysts are particularly challenging. An astute colleague, noting that candidates may not anticipate or experience a "normal" termination because they expect to work with their analysts in other roles after ending treatment, wonders whether this fact interferes with their working through their idealizing transferences. Questions for supervisors that come up in this area include: How should I deal with the fact that I work differently from the patient's analyst? When my consultation is notably helpful with clinical work that has previously been constricted by the candidate's lockstep identification with a personal psychoanalyst, how should I respond to the disillusionment in the query, "Why hasn't my own analyst been doing this?!" I do not have answers to all these questions; how to address them depends upon the specific context. But in general, differences from the candidate's analyst can be listened for, asked about, and acknowledged, and sometimes one can suggest an explanation that avoids judgments of better and worse.

Not all such differences involve disparities in theoretical orientation. For example, a candidate may be in an analysis that is well suited to her own high-functioning, depressively tilted personality, yet be treating a patient in the borderline range whose themes are more paranoid or schizoid. She would have no way to know from experience that her own analyst might work quite differently with such a person. A supervisor can comment that it is a shame that we get to know how our own analyst works only with one patient: ourselves.

There is an amusing story in Abraham Kardiner's (1977) memoir of his psychoanalysis with Freud. Kardiner, an American cultural anthropologist, learned from James Strachey, who was seeing Freud at the same time, that Freud behaved quite differently with Strachey. He reportedly said little until toward the end of the hour, when he would make a brilliant one-line interpretation. In Kardiner's own sessions, Freud was conversational, sometimes offered advice, and swapped Jewish jokes. Kardiner worried that with himself, Freud was only going through the motions. He assumed he was being treated this way because he was American (Freud was famously critical of the naive bravado and commercialism of the United States). When he voiced his complaint, Freud explained that he was adapting to Strachey's quite different personality, not giving Kardiner second-rate treatment.

Other questions that arise in supervising institute candidates concern the mentor's own psychology: What are my dynamics with respect to the supervisee's analyst? What if he or she has a powerful position in the institute? Can I present an alternative perspective without worrying about being devalued or suffering painful political consequences? What if the analyst and I are on opposing sides of a political issue important to candidates? How does our divergence affect the supervisee? Not wanting to interfere with a candidate's analysis is a worthy concern, but should not silence our own voices nor get in the way of inviting the candidate's reflections. Again, answers to such questions are elusive and contextual, but the process of being honest about differences, speculating respectfully about possible explanations for the differences, and exploring the candidate's responses to them applies here as well.

One may differ in significant ways not only from the candidate's analyst, but also from another supervisor. In fact, mature candidates deliberately expose themselves to multiple points of view, choosing mentors as exemplars of competing theoretical perspectives. When a prior or concurrent supervisor has been idealized at one's own expense, or when the candidate idealizes oneself at the expense of another supervisor, we cannot take at face value the idea that either supervisor is essentially superior. Comparative idealization and devaluation are both uncomfortable; they incite fantasies and worries about how the other analyst feels about the unfair comparison.

An important inference to draw from complications like these is that although supervisors should state confidently their own beliefs about how psychoanalytic work proceeds best, they should also avoid arrogance and preserve space for disagreement, even if the candidate is looking for a know-it-all. Speaking with the candidate's supervisor or analyst may be tempting but is unwise, at least without explicit permission, given the confidentiality constraints and the potential for infantilization in talking "behind the back" of the supervisee.

Fears about Exposure

As I noted in Chapters 4 and 5, supervisees' fears that personal information will be used in the service of negatively evaluating their progress through the institute is ubiquitous among candidates. In analytic training, even though one's own treatment tends to reduce shame about one's dynamics, such fears are amplified by the fact that psychoanalysts are legitimately expected to have a much wider, deeper knowledge of themselves than clinicians doing less ambitious therapies. Institutes expect their candidates to probe their own psyches as fully as possible in both treatment and supervision; the benefits of doing so are abundant (see Cucco, 2020). In Chapter 5, I stressed my carefulness not to intrude on the private mental spaces of novice therapists. In supervising prospective analysts, in contrast, I expect openness about countertransference reactions, personality traits, possible blind spots, trauma, and other areas that might limit the depth to which an analysis could go. I often have to articulate this difference to supervisees in institutes, as some expect it, and some do not. Helping supervisees be comfortable with a high degree of professional intimacy is challenging. Needless to say, to earn their trust, one must be a paragon of trustworthiness.

A friend of mine who devoted 15 years to being dean of students at an analytic institute tells me she thinks the hardest task of supervisors is persuading candidates, who are inevitably ambivalent about what they expose, that personal disclosures in supervision are safely confidential and will not affect their standing in the training program. Although it is true that supervisors in analytic institutes must evaluate the work of the candidates they mentor, they are rarely as critical as their supervisees imagine. As supervisors, we appreciate that we all have dynamics, vulnerabilities, and intense countertransference reactions, and that most of us were originally attracted to our field because of histories of personal suffering. And in this business, we become very good at keeping secrets. I was astonished, when I was diagnosed with breast cancer many years ago, that although most of my analytic colleagues knew about my condition, and many had close, collegial relationships with analysands of mine who were in training at the institute, none of the candidates in treatment with me heard about the diagnosis through the institute grapevine. This respect for my own choice about when to tell my patients was moving to me.

Where to draw the line between supervision and treatment is the recurrent question that institute supervisors bring up when they compare notes on how much personal disclosure they should be eliciting from supervisees. We do not want to infringe on their analyst's role, but we do want candidates to understand the myriad ways in which their personalities, dynamics, histories, and countertransferences affect their work. The easy answer to the question of the "line" is that whereas personal analysis is freely associative in all directions, supervisory exploration always returns to the patient in treatment. Everything supervisees tell us about their own psychologies should be bent to the task of helping them with clients.

When a candidate seems to be using a supervisor as an analyst, raising issues beyond a clinical focus, he or she should be encouraged to take them up in treatment—not because they are forbidden territory or upsetting to the supervisor, but because it is part of the supervisor's job to discourage splitting. It is rarely okay to know something that has been kept from the analyst. Now that our field has acknowledged how interpenetrating our psychologies inevitably are in any relationship, our understandings about line drawing have gone well beyond the naïve assumption that the analyst's or supervisor's psychology is isolatable from the relational matrix. I am probably not alone in wishing that "the line" between institute supervision and personal analysis was as easy to observe in practice as it is conceptually.

Returning to the question of candidates' worries about the implications of self-exposure in supervision for their progress through the institute, I suspect that the best antidote to such anxieties is an overall experience of integrity in the training program. In a well-functioning organization, what influences the evaluative process should be a student's demonstration of competence (or lack of it), not whether he or she has a trauma history or has struggled with an addiction or feels hatred toward a patient in the clinical moment. Any evidence that other factors are involved will become institute lore and undermine the possibility of a culture of reasonable trust.

If the supervisory relationship is not sufficiently boundaried, the supervisee's fears of exposure are eminently reasonable (see Dulchin & Segal, 1982a, 1982b). In such situations, before institute authorities can legitimately attribute candidates' inhibitions in supervision to their internal conflicts, there is a systemic problem that needs to be addressed. There have been a few infamous instances in which a candidate's privacy was not respected (e.g., Shevrin, 1981), and such crimes have had predictably damaging effects on everyone involved. Even small violations of confidences shared in the supervisor–supervisory relationship can become legendary among candidates, contributing to an unsafe atmosphere. I have made my own mistakes in this territory and speak not from a moral high ground but from painful experience and regret.

Learning is greatly enhanced in an institute, and many problems I mention in this chapter are reduced when senior analysts expose to their community the details of their treatments with patients, pointing out clinical choice points and possible ways of responding, describing countertransference reactions and enactments, and commenting on their own uncertainties and mistakes. A culture of transparency supports more realistic identifications, mutual respect, and the integration of theory with practice. But because training analysts treat candidates, and candidates often become well acquainted with each other, much clinical work cannot be shared without taking the risk that a patient, however scrupulously disguised, will be recognizable to someone in the audience.

Naturally, candidates tend to be hyperalert to this possibility. Some senior analysts have used this fact to justify refusing to present cases. A better solution to their dilemma would be that anyone in a supervisory role should treat a portion of clients who have nothing to do with the institute or the profession of psychotherapy.

Confidentiality is hard enough to protect even when one is fastidious. As I mentioned in Chapter 5, I routinely ask students in my Rutgers supervision group to inform me privately about anyone they know whom I have either treated or supervised, so that I will not use that person's intimate material didactically. Almost every year at least one member knows someone I have worked with. The connection typically surprises me. Once I was presenting a case in Australia, congratulating myself for having disguised the client well even so far from home, and an audience member with a connection to the United States identified the person on the basis of her dynamics.

In surveying a general population of psychotherapy trainees, Ladany and colleagues (1996) found that 97.2% (!) had withheld information from their supervisors. Undisclosed information included negative reactions to the supervisor, personal issues, clinical mistakes, concerns about evaluation, and countertransference reactions (see Coburn, 2001). This percentage may be lower among candidates in analytic institutes, at least in recent years, because since the time of that study, there has been considerable progress in normalizing countertransference disclosure (Cabaniss et al., 2001). But candidates have other motives for being careful about what they expose, because they typically hope to get referrals from supervisors, and unlike trainees in earlier stages of their career, referrals can be obtained right away if they are well regarded. The implications of these observations are clear: Supervisors must work hard to make candidates feel safe enough to speak openly, especially about any negative reactions to the supervision itself.

Another discipline we need to adopt is an avoidance of interpretive assumptions about the motivations for candidates' behaviors. As with patients, instead of regarding others' dynamics as self-evident, we need to open areas for exploration and clarification. A friend of mine remembers her humiliation about having turned on the air conditioner in her supervisor's waiting room. It was a hot summer day, and she had arrived early. At that time in her life, overheating caused her debilitating menopausal hot flashes. When the supervisor emerged from his office, he criticized her for having taken the liberty to operate the air conditioner without his permission, implying that her action arose from a sense of narcissistic entitlement. In a paralysis of shock, and keenly aware of the importance of his good opinion, she meekly apologized, never contradicted his interpretation, and simply tried from then on to demonstrate her lack of pathological entitlement.

Here is another instance of nondisclosure by an analytic candidate sensitive to keeping a supervisor's good opinion. A colleague of mine was grateful to his institute supervisor for seeing him at a low fee and in a convenient place that would minimize his travel during the demanding years of his early medical career. The location selected by the supervisor was a busy café. My colleague did not feel it was a safe place to talk openly about either his patient or himself, but he felt he had to accept his mentor's suggestion. Because the supervising analyst was generously extending himself, he felt it would not reflect well on him to speak up about his reservations; he might seem ungrateful for the supervisor's efforts to make his life easier. He settled for a muted, more or less constrained supervisory experience.

In Chapter 1, I emphasized the frame and the need to address boundaries explicitly with supervisees. In analytic institutes, the frame is particularly critical, both as a protection for the candidate and as a model for prospective analysts' future work with patients who test boundaries. Supervisors cannot expect that candidates will conclude from their obvious good intentions that, when asked for their evaluation of the candidate's progress, they will not be honest and forthcoming. Nor can they assume that supervisees are willing to take the risk of injuring their mentors' narcissism by expressing negative reactions to the style or content of their supervision. I remember an institute candidate who spoke with me after ending with a previous control supervisor because "his grandiosity was unbearable." She had never said a word to him about her discomfort.

As supervisors in institutes, we must be explicit about what will be shared (information about how the supervisee works with patients, keeps relevant records, cooperates with institute requirements, relates to other professionals, and responds to supervision) and what will be kept confidential (everything else). In addition to appreciating our supervisory hours as a welcome retreat from the emotional torments of in-depth clinical work, we need to make space for negative experience. We must consistently ask supervisees about areas of possible disagreement and criticism and check in periodically on their sense of safety. In other words, we must practice what we preach, demonstrating openness to the criticism and ambivalence that we expect, and train students to endure, in psychoanalytic therapies. Although I do not think that there is a need in analytic institutes for written consent to supervision, verbal consent about what is permissible to say and what is safely confidential is central to the supervisory alliance.

Potential Consequences of Supervisors' Disclosures

A related problem of institute training concerns what supervisors expose, and to whom. As I noted in previous chapters, my own tendency toward self-disclosure has proven over the years to be useful in helping graduate students feel better about their own dynamics as they surface in their work with patients. Similarly, with non-candidate professionals with whom I consult on a reciprocal basis (they pay me for the consultation; I give advice that they can take or leave), and with whom I do not live in the fishbowl of an analytic institute, I have no reluctance to talk about my mistakes and difficulties. Like my graduate students, such consultees report that knowledge of my own struggles can support their emotional honesty and self-acceptance. But an institute environment, even a healthy one, makes such disclosures more hazardous.

My graduate students' transferences toward me tend to be uncomplicated, partly because I do not occupy significant overlapping roles in their training program. Licensed practitioners with whom I consult tend to have mild transferences to me, as they are past the point of needing to idealize in intense ways. But the context of analytic training makes candidates' transferences feel much more powerful and consequential, both because of my role in evaluating them and because of the hothouse culture of the institute itself, where a disclosure to a supervisee might be shared with a classmate, who tells it to friends, until it reaches the alert ears of an analysand of mine, who then becomes excited and/or upset by the information (now often distorted, as in the game of "telephone"). I used to be critical of senior analysts for not showing more of their work or for disclosing more of their struggles, and I continue to believe that we need to do more disclosure, but I have learned to appreciate how self-protective one may become in an institute environment.

Systemic Pressures That May Contaminate Patient Care

Organizational exigencies are known to create problems for the supervision of analytic candidates (see Jaffe, 2001, on "indirect countertransferences"). An institute may require, as a prerequisite to graduating, that a candidate have seen one or more patients for a given number of sessions or have taken at least one psychoanalytic treatment through the termination phase. Such requirements, even though well-intentioned and pedagogically defensible, may subtly warp a candidate's clinical work. After years of inherently infantilizing demands to complete one training obligation after another, often well into midlife, no student of psychoanalysis, no matter how personally mature or well regarded in the role of candidate, could be impervious to incentives to graduate sooner than might otherwise be allowed.

I remember reading Firestein's (1978) book on termination and feeling a vague sense that in none of the cases he depicted had there been a truly organic, mutually agreed-upon process of termination; the endings he recounted all felt oddly forced and arbitrary. A look at his selection criteria revealed that all the treatments he described had been conducted by candidates whose institutes required them to bring a case to termination as a condition of graduating. It is not hard to conclude that the conscious and unconscious needs of the therapist could have exerted pressures on these analysands to terminate prematurely. In addition, if they were seen in the institute's low-fee clinic, their analysts were likely graduating with significant debt and hence eager to open slots in their schedules for clients who could pay regular fees. And supervisors might have their own conscious or unconscious motives to move an analysis along faster than it would evolve organically. Out of sympathy with financially strapped candidates, training analysts often provide supervision at a reduced cost, a practice that creates its own monetary incentives for bringing control cases to termination.

It is my impression that few institutes continue to make graduation conditional on bringing a case to full termination; it is now generally appreciated that such rules exert a pressure to end treatments too soon. But contaminating pressures can work in the other direction as well. Candidates surveyed by Cabaniss and Roose (1997) reported considerable anxiety that their analysands would not remain in treatment long enough for them to meet institute graduation requirements. This external reality affected them in areas such as whether to charge for missed sessions, how to schedule appointments, and what dynamics to interpret in their patients' clinical material. To me, the most arresting finding of this study was how infrequently supervisors and candidates identified together these institutional pressures and assessed their impact on the treatments of control patients. Individuals in both groups seemed to assume a posture of knowing, but not naming, that elephant in the consulting room. In a 2001 study, Cabaniss and colleagues found that despite the fact that "50 percent of candidates reported anxiety about receiving credit for cases, this was not routinely discussed in supervision, and the supervisory relationship itself was not discussed in over 50 percent of dyads" (p. 235).

It is an ethical problem if supervisors and candidates conspire, even unconsciously, to keep someone in analysis who is ready to launch, or to terminate treatment with a patient who needs more time, or to work with a training case differently than they would with a person who has less potential impact on their professional advancement. Obviously, in any clinical situation there are financial and other influences on the therapist that can compromise treatment (for example, arbitrary decisions about length and frequency imposed by third-party payers), but in institutes there are even more sources of contamination, including more subtle ones. Supervisors need to pay attention to these realities, as candidates evidently hesitate to bring them up.

The main inference I draw from scholarly research on the supervisee experience is that supervisors should raise issues of potential conflict between institute requirements and patient need, and that both parties in the supervisory relationship should face them squarely, with the aim of putting the patient's welfare ahead of the therapist's progress through the training program. The second implication of findings like those of the Cabaniss group is that candidates, supervisors, and institute authorities should consider and advocate for changes in how candidate progress is evaluated, so that the likelihood that training requirements will compromise treatment is reduced. And third, if there is no way to prevent external factors from affecting the treatment (for example, if either fixed clinic policies or dire financial straits make it impossible for the therapist to continue to see low-fee patients after graduating), supervisor and supervisee have to find ways of acknowledging these realities with patients. Many analysands worry about such factors anyway (e.g., "You don't care about me; you just need me for your training"), and some are highly attuned to their shadowy impact on the therapeutic relationship.

In addition to helping candidates address the content of this accusation by nondefensive acknowledgment (e.g., "Yes, the reason that you are getting such a good deal on an in-depth treatment is that I am in postgraduate training, and my hours with you count toward my graduation requirements"), supervisors need to help candidates investigate the meaning of comments like these. Even at the postgraduate level, clinicians can be knocked off-kilter by statements about how little they "really" care, and they can forget to explore what concern generates such assertions and to examine why that issue seems suddenly relevant, and so on. Behind complaints like these there is often a yearning for unlimited, unconditional, healing love, the fantasy of an omnipotent mother who can make everything okay if only she "gets it" about her child's bottomless need. Supervisees need to be sure they expose this wish as a universal but unrealistic desire rather than try to show the patient how much they care. Efforts to prove that their devotion to a patient goes beyond conscientious professional care will typically set them up for one regressive test after another of their love—a valuable lesson to learn when one is in training, as such tests will happen again.

One more potentially treatment-distorting pressure in analytic institutes concerns the requirement that candidates conduct a "standard," "traditional," or "classical" psychoanalysis with one or more patients. Depth-psychological treatments exert a regressive pull, which can be vital to the growth of healthier patients but disorganizing and destructive to more troubled ones. Institutes try to ensure that individuals who are accepted as candidates for intensive psychoanalysis are suited to working at high frequency and/or on the couch, and yet it is an open secret that patients initially considered good candidates for traditional treatment often turn out to be borderline, severely personality disordered, addicted, dissociative, suicidal, and even psychotic (Lauro et al., 2003). To meet the institute requirement, the candidate and supervisor may try to force the patient into the procrustean bed of the institute's favored technical approach, and sometimes they manage to make this work out (mainly because the patient can sense the analyst's determination to help), but I hope it is obvious that trying to adapt psychoanalytic treatment to the patient is preferable to trying to adapt the patient to an idealized version of psychoanalytic treatment.

For many intersecting reasons, there has been a serious decline in the number of individuals who want (or can afford) intensive and extensive psychoanalytic treatment, as well as a seeming increase in disorders (e.g., posttraumatic and addictive problems) that respond well to psychodynamic therapies but not to classical analysis (Lauro et al., 2003). These days, the majority of patients in standard treatments are probably candidates at analytic institutes. But even in the era when psychoanalysis had great social cachet, the number of "analyzable" patients was far from ideal, and many institute candidates struggled through their training trying to make their image of standard technique fit clients for whom it was not the treatment of choice (and keeping quiet about it when they made intuitively compelling and effective deviations from orthodoxy).

The problem of finding sufficient analysands for candidates in training is thus contextual and systemic. It cannot be addressed solely at the level of individual supervisor and supervisee. This is another area in which supervisors may have to press their organizations to adapt to external realities. In many institutes, the problem has been addressed by adding programs in psychodynamic therapy to the institute's training offerings (although in those cultures, traditional psychoanalysis tends to remain the more valued praxis). In some training programs, requirements involving frequency and use of the couch have been modified. Many organizational problems of psychoanalytic training remain to be solved, but in the meantime, supervisors must muddle along, remaining aware of realities that inevitably affect their work.

A Note on Unresolvable Hurt Feelings and the Supervisory Atmosphere

When I see candidates in my local analytic community in treatment, they not infrequently tell me hurtful things that colleagues or students have said about me. The "basic rule" of free association gives them no option of protecting me from such comments, even if they prefer to do so, and when they seem to be trying to keep something out of our work, I tend to sense it and urge them to push past any reluctance to speak. Reports of unflattering remarks tend to be made in the context of strong and potentially distorting transferences. As a result, I never know how accurate they are, and there is no way for me to fact-check them.

Because everything "from the couch" is confidential, I cannot do what I normally would do if I were to hear in a nonconfidential context that a friend or colleague had criticized me, namely, find an opportunity to say, "I heard that you said my judgment is poor. Is that really what you think? Can we talk about that?" Instead, I have to *contain* my feelings in an even more disciplined way than psychotherapy usually requires. I cannot "unhear" a hurtful remark, and I cannot deal explicitly with it. It can complicate my relationships in ways I can do nothing about. It is an irony of psychoanalytic practice that analysts are often prevented from doing what we help our patients to do: speak directly with people who cause them pain. Accumulations of such untreated wounds and residual grudges can have a subtle but significant impact on the atmosphere of an institute. In the role of supervisor, it is incumbent on us not to act out in any way that exacerbates this occupational hazard, such as using our supervisees to carry messages to analysts we dislike.

QUALIFICATIONS FOR PSYCHOANALYTIC SUPERVISION:
A VEXED ISSUE

In the institutes of the American Psychoanalytic Association, the status of training analyst is highly coveted. It involves a subjective selection process that has become quite controversial (Kernberg, 2014b; Kernberg & Michels, 2016). In North American institutes not affiliated with the APsaA, the more usual criterion for training analyst status is having practiced psychoanalytically for a certain number of years after graduation from a reputable institute. In some psychoanalytic training programs in Europe, notably in France, there is much less institutionalization of varying levels of supervisory responsibility. The IPA recognizes several different systems of analytic training.

There has been virtually no research—which would in any case be quite hard to design —comparing the outcomes of different training approaches. Kenneth Eisold noted in 2000 that institutionally, psychoanalysis has so far failed to assume the responsibility of studying and clarifying its own practices, and although there is more critical literature now than in 2000, his observation remains accurate: Analytic institutes have been notably resistant to having their educational practices examined empirically. There is, however, a sizeable and contentious professional literature on the question. Analytic institutes have been legitimately critiqued for a culture of charismatic authority, indoctrination, and even secret manipulation and exploitation (Kirsner, 2000). Like other organizations, they are rife with politics, and have been since the earliest machinations of Freud and his followers. Supervisors in analytic institutes need to be aware of the political currents in their environment and not take them too personally.

Many thoughtful critics within the psychoanalytic community have questioned our training models and made suggestions for improving psychoanalytic education (Arlow, 1972; Auchincloss & Michels, 2003; Balint, 1948; Berman, 2001; Bernfeld, 1962; Eisold, 2004; A. Freud, 1938; Kairys, 1964; Kernberg, 1986, 2000, 2010, 2014b; Kernberg & Michels, 2016; Reeder, 2004; Wallerstein, 2010). Research on the experience of psychoanalytic supervision from the trainees' point of view is only in its infancy. In one of the small number of studies on candidates' reports, Cabaniss and colleagues (2001) found striking disagreements between supervisees and supervisors about the supervisor's role, about evaluation, about what is most useful to candidates, and about the relationship between supervision and progression to graduation.

A HYPOTHESIS ABOUT CULTURES OF ENMESHMENT

I suspect that the ease of supervision in psychoanalytic institutes, or the comfort of both parties and the effectiveness of the supervisory process, is inversely proportional to the extent that the organization is "incestuous"; that is, the more overlap the institute has in roles and relationships, the harder the job of supervisor. This is a testable hypothesis, which I hope will someday be empirically investigated. Smaller institutes, and those providing the only analytic training in their geographical area, may be particularly subject to stresses on supervisors that involve basic boundary issues. Supervision in institutes that requires candidates to be analyzed and supervised by one of their own senior members may be particularly challenging. Such requirements are typically defended by institute authorities as ensuring "high standards" of treatment and education; after all, the analyst and supervisor have both been thoroughly vetted by the organization. But it is hard to overlook the self-interest in such rules, which make it possible for senior analysts to have a reliable and self-renewing stream of customers. And their impact can be deadening.

The most positive experiences I have had as an institute supervisor have been with the National Training Program (NTP) of the National Institute for the Psychotherapies (NIP). This 4-year "distant learner" program serves aspiring psychoanalysts who prefer not to get training where they live or work or whose home city lacks an institute. They come to New York City for six intensive weekends of course work per year and obtain their personal analysis and supervision either in their own community or remotely. NTP's criteria for being a training analyst (*nipinst.org*, August 13, 2020) are (1) graduation from a "postgraduate psychoanalytic training program or its equivalent" at least 5 years previously and (2) the approval of their training committee. Supervisors ("consultants") must be "approved of or affiliated with" NIP.

These clear-cut standards give candidates ample latitude and minimize the emotional and political complexity common to small local institutes, where one's supervisor is inevitably the analyst of a classmate, is at odds with one's favorite teacher, or sits on a committee with the candidate as a student representative. NTP's long-distance arrangements seem to make analysts in training more closely bonded as a class, less defensive about their own dynamics, and less competitive with one another for the same scarce human resources. Their interactions lack the acute self-consciousness that can permeate more localized institute settings even when everyone is being as respectful of boundaries as possible.

Although I have not had an NTP candidate in analysis, I assume the distance-learning model also reduces the frequency with which analysts and supervisors suffer from reports of painful criticisms from friends and colleagues.

If I am right that supervisory complications in analytic communities are inversely proportional to role overlap, then the common rule that a candidate's personal analyst must be a member of the institute should be challenged. Personal treatment is much cleaner and more meaningful for those who experience the privacy that comes with having an analyst outside their community. And because of the "cross-fertilization" it offers, analyses of candidates by someone outside the institute may benefit both the training analyst and the home institute. Enmeshment and the resulting anxiety about privacy may be the main sources of the conventional lore in traditional American institutes that one undergoes one analysis "for the institute" and one "for me" (Wallerstein, 2010, p. 932).

Perhaps even more consequentially, it has always seemed crazy to me that people who are willing to make the sacrifices necessary to pursue analytic training, and who have often developed that interest because of a positive experience in psychoanalysis, should be expected to end treatment summarily with a professional who has been deeply helpful to them and start over with someone else. This seems not only unfair to them and to their analyst but also self-defeating for institutes. They pay a high long-term price for the narcissistic and economic rewards of monopolizing the candidate market in their area.

I know of several talented therapists who decided not to pursue analytic training because they knew they would be asked to abandon their perfectly good personal treatment. In fact, I made a comparable decision myself. In the mid-1970s, my husband Carey was offered an attractive professorship at Johns Hopkins University in Maryland. I was in training in New York at the time but, having terminated my personal analysis of several years, was willing to move if the Baltimore institute would accept me as a candidate. My interviewer there stated that even though I was not a physician, I was a strong applicant. But then she added that "of course" I would have to get a new analyst.

I was naïve about psychoanalytic politics at the time and asked why, since my NPAP analyst and I had had a very successful experience. "Your analyst isn't a member of the American Psychoanalytic Association," she explained. She went on to say that there was no way he would be accepted either. "But he was trained by Theodor Reik, who was trained by Freud." No matter. Then she added, "But don't worry, analysis with another person would only be a training analysis. You just have to log the hours." I was appalled by her concept of a *pro forma* analysis, and that was the end of the Johns Hopkins option. But evidently, the fact that the "didactic" analysis was not a "real" analysis was common knowledge in the medical psychoanalytic culture of that period, and according to recent critics of the training analyst system, there are institutes where it still is (Kernberg & Michels, 2016; Wallerstein, 2010).

EVALUATION

Except in a few places in the United States where psychoanalysis is licensed as a separate profession (that is, where becoming an analyst does not require prior credentialing in a helping profession and where psychoanalysis has the legal status of a freestanding profession), candidates in analytic institutes can already practice independently. This reality lifts a burden from their supervisors, who then do not have to report to external licensing boards and regulatory bodies about their mentee's suitability to be a therapist. But they do have to weigh in on how well each supervisee is mastering critical analytic theory, research, and clinical writing. They are also expected to comment on the degree to which a candidate has assimilated a psychoanalytic identity (see Nagell et al., 2014) and has basic psychoanalytic clinical competence (Killingmo, Varvin, & Strømme, 2014; Strømme, 2014). Supervisors may also have to assess whether the candidate has any personality tendencies that might compromise more ambitious psychoanalytic treatments even though they may not be a problem in other assessment, counseling, or clinical work.

In psychotherapy, the therapeutic alliance depends on certain elements: agreement about the problem being addressed, some degree of mutual understanding about the approach to be used to improve the situation, clarity about the respective tasks of the patient and clinician, and concurrence about what will constitute evidence of the therapy's eventual success. In analytic institutes, there is little analogous clarity about the elements of the supervisory alliance. Supervisors tend to address the first three aspects according to their own preferences (what are the areas the mentor and mentee determine as needing work, how will the supervision sessions be structured, and what is the role of each party). Supervisors have considerable latitude, for example, in their individual preferences about working from process notes, videotapes, or verbal reports. Supervisees need to be encouraged to represent their own preferences because they evidently tend to defer rather than to negotiate.

The third area, the nature of evidence that a candidate has made significant progress toward psychoanalytic competence, requires institutes and general policies to be clearer at a systems level. The absence of such clarity may be a key source of the inconsistencies found by Cabaniss and colleagues (2001).

Because of the substantial differences in patients with respect to what moves the analytic process along, and because of the pluralism in the field, this process is inherently vexed and inevitably subjective (see Kantrowitz, 2002). To my knowledge, although there have been recommendations for a more objective evaluation of analytic competence, none of these have been widely adopted. It remains the case that in most analytic training, the criteria for graduation tend to be vague and open to varying interpretations (see Vaughan, Spitzer, Davies, & Roose, 1997), and the subjectivity in the evaluation process is not counterbalanced by objective criteria (Kernberg & Michels, 2016).

The best advice I can give supervisors involves two areas. First, we need to keep all our comments, especially our negative evaluations, tied tightly to the supervisee's behavior rather than giving our diagnostic impressions of the supervisee. Instead of saying, "I think Sally's narcissism is still a problem," we could say, "I am concerned about the degree to which Sally talks about herself with patients. I think it distracts them from going deeper into their own thoughts and feelings." Instead of saying, "David sometimes behaves masochistically with patients," one could say, "There have been several instances in which David seemed to have trouble setting limits, and patients have responded with regressive behavior and escalating demands." Promiscuous diagnosing is a plague at many analytic institutes.

Second, we need to share our evaluative thoughts (tactfully) with our supervisees. The supervisory relationship needs to be mined for all the ways it picks up the relational patterns of the candidate. Although supervising analysts have a responsibility to own their contributions to any enactments, they still have the job of eventually evaluating a separate person. Nothing of an evaluative nature that arises at the end of a candidate's formal training should be a surprise. Rationalizing lack of criticism as protective seems to me an insult to the capable adults who seek our mentorship.

The most painful situation for an institute supervisor is fortunately rare: the candidate who simply fails to "get" other people. Theodor Reik observed in 1948 (p. 3) that the gift for psychological observation is "as inborn as a musical sense or a mathematical talent. Where it is not present, nothing—not even courses, lectures, and seminars—will produce it." This reality has not changed since 1948. Although the general loss of the prestige of psychoanalysis may have led to fewer applications of untalented candidates (these days, most people who apply for institute training are not seeking professional advancement per se; they have a genuine feel for the work), every few years one encounters a candidate who has a tin ear instead of a "third ear."

Even though a supervisor's assessment is unlikely to destroy one's entire career in mental health (because of the credential the clinician had when applying for postgraduate training), an institute candidate invests immense amounts of time, money, and emotion into becoming an analyst. For narcissistic reasons, and because of the potential loss of a valued community, to be told that one lacks the aptitude for in-depth psychoanalytic work can be psychologically devastating. Nevertheless, when no amount of course work, supervision, and personal analysis has improved a candidate's ability to mentalize others, a supervisor has to say so. This situation is simply excruciating, and I have no idea how to make it less so. More than one analyst has confessed to me that they had felt morally bound to tell the truth about an untalented trainee at evaluation meetings but were relieved when colleagues outvoted them.

There is so much variation in how institutes assess mature psychoanalytic competence that it is hard to generalize about the supervisor's role in preparing the candidate. I know of a few cases in which a person has gone through the final evaluation process several times; eventually the candidate was given what I have heard called a "compassionate graduation." Does this mean we are graduating people who should not be psychoanalysts? Or does it mean that the skills involved in making an impressive case presentation are significantly different from the skills required to be a good analyst? A member of one of my consultation groups seemed to me an exemplary analyst, but his long-standing, trauma-based stage fright greatly compromised his capacity to represent himself publicly to others. I found myself thinking that the amount of rehearsal, exposure, yoga, mindfulness practice, and beta blockers that went into his preparations for his final case presentation could have been much better spent on immersion in psychoanalytic ideas.

I was interested to learn recently that my local institute (CPPNJ) has changed the rules for the final case papers and presentations. Readiness to gradate is determined by prior evaluation by teachers and supervisors. Although members of the final case committee give feedback to the graduating analyst, it is only advisory. Institute leaders made this change because previously candidates might be failed or be given unexpected conditions to meet before getting a diploma, on the basis of criticisms they had never heard before. The frequency with which this practice occurred had created a culture of paranoid anxiety about this ultimate rite of passage (cf. Kernberg, 1986, 1996).

CPPNJ thus recast the final case paper and presentation rules as the consequence rather than the verification of a readiness to graduate and put more onus on supervisors and teachers to evaluate candidates along the way. (This obligation can also include the painful task of persuading a student to delay graduation.) Interestingly, candidates continue to report a dread of the ritual marking the end of their formal training. Institute leaders hope such apprehensions are less paranoid now. They would like to understand them as normal worries about looking competent, magnified by the separation anxiety inherent in an event symbolizing a new level of professional adulthood. But everyone in the institute is still evaluating the effects of the change.

ON PREPARING CANDIDATES FOR INSTITUTE SUPERVISION

It is still relatively uncommon for institutes to offer courses *in supervision* to their candidates. Those of us of a certain age learned it, for better or worse, from being supervised ourselves. That dearth of classes in the dynamics and techniques of supervision is thankfully beginning to change. There is now a robust-enough literature on psychoanalytic supervision to design several syllabi, and some institutes have done so. My own preference for how to structure a course in supervision would be for advanced candidates in institutes to be expected to supervise beginning analytic candidates, and for these supervisors-in-training to meet in a confidential course in which they read clinical and empirical writings on supervision and regularly present supervisory problems to one another.

One goal such a course could not achieve is a goal that this chapter cannot achieve, either: the restructuring of analytic training so that it is less reflective of old-boy-network group dynamics, less paranoiagenic, and more supportive of the creativity, maturity, and diversity of candidates. The problem of training people in a field where there is so little agreement on what constitutes competence in its own practice remains. The good news, however, is that analysts are now engaged in a lively conversation about how to approach these long-standing problems (Fonagy & Allison, 2016; Kernberg & Michels, 2016; Layton, 2016; Levy, 2016; McWilliams, 2016; Seligman, 2016). Recently, the Columbia University Center for Psychoanalytic Training and Research has adopted major changes in training to address the problems I depict (Richardson, Cabaniss, Halperin, Vaughan, & Cherry, 2020).

CONCLUDING COMMENTS

In this chapter, I have discussed both satisfactions and dissatisfactions of mentoring candidates in analytic institutes. The former are substantial, but so are the latter, which include problems of psychoanalytic identity, consequences of idealization and devaluation, fears about possible consequences of self-exposure, inhibitions on supervisors' disclosures, contaminations of patient care by training requirements, and other systemic stresses. I have also commented about problems with institute evaluation processes. Finally, I have noted the need for, and increasing provision of, courses in supervision for analytic candidates and made a suggestion about how they might be organized.

After digesting my list of criticisms of analytic training programs, a reader might conclude that I find postgraduate psychoanalytic education, or at least supervising in institutes, more trouble than it is worth. That is emphatically not the case. For all its complications and frustrations, I found my own analytic training consistently stimulating intellectually and fulfilling emotionally. The warmth and integrity of those with whom I studied became integral to my own psychoanalytic identity. I continue to appreciate how they coped gracefully with a complicated training environment and supported my sense of safety, self-esteem, and adulthood despite many competing pressures. I have tried to do the same. The psychoanalytic communities with which I have been connected remain a vital part of my life. It has been a privilege to supervise and consult with candidates going through the unique stresses and rewards of analytic training.

Chapter Eight

■   ■   ■   ■

Individual Differences and Specific Supervisory Challenges

Empirical studies of supervision suggest that the supervisory alliance is as central to clinical maturation as the therapeutic alliance is to therapeutic progress (Gard & Lewis, 2008; Watkins, 2015b). In the role of clinical mentor, one quickly learns that each supervisory dyad is as individual as each therapy dyad, and that making adaptations to a unique supervisee has a lot in common with making adaptations to a unique patient.

There has been surprisingly little research on how therapists' unique personalities affect their work or relate to supervision, beyond the overall evidence for the value of general qualities, such as empathy, the ability to listen, and genuine curiosity (see Ackerman & Hilsenroth, 2003). In an important study of therapists' perceptions of the effects of their personal issues on their clinical work, Bernhardt, Nissen-Lie, Moltu, McLeod, and Råbu (2019) supported the value of attention to this area, explored positive and negative implications of therapist individuality (especially wounded-healer themes), and concluded that clinicians' vulnerability should be worked with rather than "resolved." This chapter addresses several specific areas of individual variability as they might affect supervisor and supervisee, both individually and in the co-constructed supervisory relationship.

For many years I have been part of a group of amateur singers. Our teacher has a genius for knowing, after listening to a single solo performance, exactly how to help the singer do it better the next time. We never know if he will focus on pitch, tempo, breath control, voice placement, phrasing, emotional interpretation, body language, or communication with the audience, but once he hears one of us sing, he has a knack for zeroing in on precisely the issue that, in the moment, we are capable of improving. Psychotherapy supervision is a lot like that process: the sensitive teaching of an art or skill, informed by what the apprentice artist is currently capable of correcting, adjusting, or refining. But unlike the training of singers, clinical supervision is complicated by the fact that supervisory responsibilities extend beyond the supervised therapist. The obligation to do right by each supervisee's patients is a critical constraint on the general directive to "start where the person is."

My experiences of engagement with that complication are what prompted my writing this chapter. Some therapists practically inhale supervision; they seem to have no difficulty internalizing and applying what a more seasoned colleague recommends. Naturally inquisitive and flexible people can readily assimilate guidance and adapt it to their own style with patients. Fortunately, most of my experiences as a supervisor have been with clinicians who enjoy supervision and are eager to learn as much as they can. Some therapists, however, seem to resist learning; their responses to supervision resemble those of patients whose anxieties about change keep them stuck in a defensive stance. Sometimes such resistances arise because of an unfortunate fit between supervisor and supervisee, and sometimes they are primarily characterological; either way, they complicate the educational process. It can be just as hard to repair a supervisory stalemate as it is to move past a clinical impasse. Often, we cannot help our trainees toward professional mastery any faster than we can help our patients toward personal maturity.

SOME RELEVANT PERSONALITY CONFIGURATIONS

When a supervisee cannot find internally the understanding and autonomy that will allow him or her to absorb a mentor's thinking and put supervisory recommendations into practice, or to initiate a problem-solving discussion that can resolve differences of perspective, supervisors may have to insist, out of concern for the patient, that the clinician behave in ways that go beyond what comes naturally or easily to that person. That extra burden on the supervisory alliance creates tensions that vary with the unique psychologies of both parties. In this section I explore several dynamics that can tax the supervisory dyad, along with some thoughts about ways to reduce the problems associated with them.

My own psychology is predominantly hysterical and depressive (I do not suffer from hysterical symptoms or clinical depression, but my personality is organized by dynamics that are prominent in those conditions). In the supervisory examples I provide here from my own experience, these tendencies may be evident. Because they derive from the interaction between my own dynamics and those of the people I consult with, my recommendations will have to be adapted to the work of supervisors with different personality inclinations, who may need to find ways of approaching resistances and resolving interpersonal impasses with supervisees that comport better with their own personalities.

Depressive and Masochistic Dynamics in Supervision

As I noted in previous chapters, the psychologies of psychotherapists, presumably both supervisors and supervisees, are frequently infused with depressive and/or self-defeating dynamics (Hyde, 2009). These include introjective processes and reaction formations against one's aggressive potentials that manifest themselves in deep-rooted tendencies toward guilt, self-reproach, and an internal pressure to prioritize the needs and perspectives of others at the expense of those of the self (Campos, 2013; Huprich, 1998, 2014; McWilliams, 2011; Shedler & Westen, 2004). Given the prevalence of a depressive–masochistic orientation (Kernberg, 1988) among therapists, the most common supervisory dyad may consist of a characterologically depressive mentor and a depressively organized mentee.

In Chapter 4, I talked about the value of interpreting a clinician's masochistic defenses when they appear in supervision in the form of automatic self-criticism unconsciously intended to preempt the supervisor's anticipated disapproval. That phenomenon is a specific, situationally triggered expression of self-attacking dynamics that can often be named, contextualized, and transcended. But there are more general, less visible features of depressive and self-defeating psychology that may need supervisory attention, including difficulty in setting limits with patients, difficulty in admitting differences of opinion with supervisors, tendencies to be ingratiating, tendencies to "take care of" the other's self-esteem at the price of inauthenticity, an inability to identify or address instances of aggression in patients or the self, and so on.

The most problematic aspect of working with a depressively inclined supervisee, especially if the supervisor shares a depressive tilt, may be a tendency to be so concerned with the supervisee's narcissistic equilibrium that one withholds legitimate criticism of the person's work. In a complementary dynamic, for a supervisee who is depressive, the automatic inclination to support the self-esteem of the supervisor can preclude the exploration of differences of perspective and can thereby limit learning. Depressive individuals tend to idealize and take care of people they depend on. Unlike people with more narcissistic psychologies, who idealize in an empty way ("My doctor is the best in the country!" or "That is just brilliant!"), depressive people idealize based on real qualities in the other. In supervision, they appreciate their mentor's knowledge, kindness, and good intentions.

Because of these personality patterns, depressive therapists are a delight to supervise; they are earnest and conscientious, and they work hard to understand a supervisor's perspective and follow his or her advice. But mentors of supervisees with depressive psychologies have to keep an eye on the possibility that they are withholding negative feedback that could improve their collaboration in supervision or even their work with patients. Making a depressively organized clinician feel safe enough to express disagreement or criticism is a vital contribution to the person's professional development. It is a curse of therapists to be so oriented toward empathy that we fail to stand back, notice what is problematic, and call out what needs to be addressed.

An important aspect of the clinical role, as every supervisee unhappily learns, is how to impart unwelcome information. The art of telling it like it is without triggering a patient's tendency to feel personally attacked cannot be developed if one has too great a reluctance to be the bearer of bad news. Therapists learn how to be forthright with their patients by witnessing a supervisor's frankness about what both parties might prefer to ignore. To learn to tolerate the devaluation with which many prospective patients will approach them, depressively inclined clinicians need help with keeping their self-esteem intact even when their mistakes are pointed out. If they do not get used to confrontation in the context of overall support, they will have trouble tolerating negative transferences and will be inauthentically sympathetic with patients in hostile states of mind, who will then feel frustrated that their own message of negativity is not getting through, and may escalate to ensure that it does.

There are additional professional reasons to help these supervisees get used to constructive criticism. To survive in our profession, clinicians need to know that even intense disagreements are not always equivalent to ad hominem attacks. In the absence of evidence of a personal vendetta, critical comments should not be taken personally. Learning to accept criticism without undue defensiveness requires disciplined practice. Practitioners whose skin is too thin to endure negative feedback will not likely take the risk of future engagement in critically important arguments about such issues as mental health policy, standards for psychotherapy training, and clinical guidelines. In addition, they are unlikely to submit their ideas to journal editors and then benefit from the critiques of peer reviewers who are sometimes less than tactful.

Supervisors with core depressive dynamics tend to project them on to supervisees whether or not a particular clinician's psychology is depressive. The most cringe-worthy lapse in my supervisory career occurred during my brief individual work with a practitioner who (fortunately) decided to change his profession as soon as he ran into the emotional stresses of clinical work. He was a heterosexual man treating an attractive female heterosexual patient for posttraumatic symptoms related to childhood sexual abuse. In the face of her relentless pleas for a hug, he had capitulated, taken her into his arms, and found himself getting an erection. In telling me about the incident, he complained about her seductive appearance and unceasing pressure on him. He seemed to have no sense of his own culpability in the enactment.

If I had heard an account like this from someone else, I would have been quite judgmental. But I was fond of this man, who was new to the field and unfamiliar with handling the erotic countertransferences that often permeate work with patients who have been sexually traumatized. My initial response to his story was sympathy with his mental state. I think I sensed also that his feelings would be hurt if I called him out on his ethical violation. Although I knew he had made a serious error, transgressing normal clinical boundaries in ways all too reminiscent of the patient's previous molesters, I found myself colluding with his pathologizing her and normalizing his own behavior.

It was my good luck that in addition to being in individual supervision, this man was in one of my consultation groups. When he told the story there, his colleagues immediately faulted him for his bad judgment and took me to task for my tacit acceptance of the narrative that he had been the victim of the patient rather than the one who overstepped boundaries. Instead of supporting a shift to Klein's (1946) depressive position, in which he could have mentalized his client more compassionately, I had indeed implicitly supported his remaining in the paranoid–schizoid state of blaming her. This leads me to the next topic.

Paranoid Dynamics in Supervision

Supervisors should be aware of the possibility that paranoid reactions during training may reflect situational rather than characterological dynamics. As I noted in Chapter 7, organizations and programs can create paranoid environments, especially when rules and expectations are not explicit and transparent. Even in the absence of systemic sources, paranoia is a common response to being observed and evaluated; supervisors may themselves suffer mild paranoia when students will be formally evaluating them, when a faculty is considering them for a regular position, or when an institute is assessing their suitability to be a training analyst. In its situational versions, paranoia is unremarkable in supervision.

In the realm of personality dynamics, in contrast, although individuals who are attracted to being therapists seldom have a visibly paranoid personality organization, I have known a few (both supervisors and supervisees) who described themselves as characterologically paranoid or whose personality could be inferred to be in that territory. Because supervising in the context of paranoid dynamics is challenging and sometimes counterintuitive, this section is somewhat lengthy. I have supervised or consulted with only a few individuals with paranoid personality styles, and so I offer the following ideas tentatively.

I should specify first I am not using the term "paranoia" in the descriptive DSM sense as referring to unreasonable suspiciousness or fearfulness. One can be unrealistically fearful based on many dynamics (phobic or posttraumatic processes, for example). The paranoid process as it has specifically been theorized in the analytic literature (e.g., Auchincloss & Weiss, 1992; Freud, 1896, 1911b; Meissner, 1978; Oldham & Bone, 1997; Shapiro, 1965) involves disavowing a disturbing internal state (e.g., anger, desire, vulnerability, shame, envy) and projecting it onto others, who are then seen as manifesting the disowned state that has been projected. What is internal and unacceptable becomes external and often threatening. Paranoid inclinations in a growing child can be fueled by repeated experiences of humiliation (Garfield & Havens, 1991; Shengold, 1989) and/or gaslighting (Calef & Weinshel, 1981), whether from the child's family or peers, or through simply the subjective experience of falling short of one's own black-or-white standards of goodness. In the paranoid process, anything potentially humiliating risks being an experience of retraumatization and so becomes denied and projected.

Consequently, the primary concern of the supervisor working with a paranoid supervisee should be to relate to the therapist as a human equal and to avoid shaming or talking down to him or her. Paranoid individuals are exquisitely sensitive to being patronized or humored rather than being approached with respect. They are not afraid of differences of opinion—unlike more depressive people, they tend to be reassured of someone's honesty and lack of manipulativeness when the person is willing to "tell it like it is"—but when a difference of opinion or a suggestion for change is expressed in ways that feel humiliating to the supervisee, rigid defenses that interfere with subsequent learning can arise.

Especially if their history involved gaslighting, paranoid people require an exceedingly demanding level of honesty in their mentors. They often notice characteristics of the supervisor that are true and perhaps unremarkable, but to which they ascribe personal and negative implications. That is, they get the feeling or attitude right but the interpretation wrong. One has to be alert to the possibility of their taking personally and critically some offhand or seemingly trivial remark. My own way of coping with the relational challenges posed by a mentee with significant paranoia, once the clinician and I have a good alliance, is to be (1) as honest as I am capable of being and (2) more than typically self-disclosing, especially about my uncertainties and shortcomings. I do this in a matter-of-fact way, as if limitation is to be expected. At the same time, I do not minimize my competence and confidence as a therapist. I take this stance of demonstrated humility combined with basic self-trust for several reasons.

First, I hope that my disclosures of my own mistakes and failings will contribute to reducing paranoid–schizoid dichotomies (e.g., good versus bad technique, competent versus incompetent intervention, ethical versus unethical practice), nudging the therapist toward the capacity to mentalize by example alone, without pointing to limitations in the trainee that would be humiliating and therefore disorganizing. Trying to expand the space for thinking about better and worse, appreciating paradox, understanding trade-offs, and other elements of the complexity of psychotherapy, is particularly valuable for clinicians with paranoid tendencies. In addressing this area using the example of my own behavior without critical or interpretive commentary, I try to reduce the supervisee's overall vulnerability to humiliation about inevitable fallibility.

Second, rather than trying to direct a paranoid-inclined person's attention to his or her disavowing and projective defenses, which could either be rejected defensively or experienced as shameful, I am hoping that the exposure of mental states in myself that are often viewed negatively will detoxify the thoughts, feelings, and fantasies that instigate the person's need to disavow and project. For example, with one supervisee

who tended to deny his own reactiveness to situations of loss and separation and instead look for people to blame for his distress, I mentioned
matter-of-factly, in connection with the dynamics of one of his patients,
my own anxious and depressive reactions to separations, giving a couple
of examples. I hoped that he could identify with my acknowledgment of
my own feelings about loss and move toward embracing a normal grief
reaction rather than imprisoning himself in a paranoid state of mind. If
he could do that, he could perhaps help his clients to do the same.

Third, when I am the object of criticism, either from the supervisee
or someone known to him or her, I try to model the capacity to separate
the criticism from the criticizer. I remember one somewhat paranoid
supervisee in my analytic institute who knew that I was in a political
battle with a colleague. She was astonished to learn that even though
I was fighting this man aggressively in the public realm, we continued
to enjoy a warm personal relationship. By mentioning our friendship, I
hoped to help this woman understand that differences of opinion need
not turn others into bad objects and that being friendly with people
who disagree with us, even on critical matters, does not equate with
hypocrisy.

As I have noted, people with paranoia are hyperaware of their emotional surround and frequently pick up affects accurately. Where they
get into trouble is not in what they identify but in their self-referential
interpretation of its meaning. Therapists with a paranoid streak who
cannot appreciate the difference between the person and the position
the person is taking, even at an intellectual level (and that was a clear
strain for my institute supervisee, who worried that I was naïve about
my friend's dangerousness), will be handicapped clinically. For example,
they will find it hard to work with patients who differ with them politi-
cally. They will conflate criticism with hatred. More subtly, they will
have trouble absorbing the reality that individuals who savagely condemn their caregivers also love them. Without a feel for this apparent
contradiction, they may wrongly assume that a complaining patient will
feel emotionally supported by their agreeing that some authority is a
monster; the client's defense of negligent or abusive parents will then
surprise them. They will find it hard to understand that patients who
torment a therapist with negative transferences may also have feelings of
deep attachment.

Fourth, I tend to challenge the typical paranoid confusion between
warmth and weakness. People with paranoid tendencies are often in a
terrible bind: They have unconscious anxieties that their negative feelings are powerful and dangerous, and yet at the same time, they worry

that their positive feelings (e.g., attachment, compassion, hope, trust, and enjoyment) and their more passive negative states (e.g., sadness, shame, and longing) will make them sitting ducks for someone else's abuse. They tend to equate tender feelings with fragility and naiveté. Consequently, they need a supervisor who seems solid and unintimidated and at the same time is unafraid to be moved. A mentor who is frank about vulnerability can come across as more powerful than one who denies normal dependency, emotional reactivity, and the inevitability of making mistakes. A mentor's calm acceptance of vulnerability may also reassure a paranoid supervisee that the mentor is undamaged by any hostility, aggression, envy, and other negative aspects of the supervisee's mental life; a sense of the supervisor's solidity should reduce the need to disown and project such internal states.

I remember vividly the distressed reaction of one rather paranoid supervisee when I teared up at his description of a patient's painful history. Thinking my emotional response meant that I was on the verge of emotional collapse, he was astonished when I reframed my capacity to feel compassion as a strength. I went on to say that the assumption that stoicism equals strength, or that feeling one's pain or tearing up in a session means some kind of "loss of control," reflects a limited Western mind-set. I reminded him that in many cultures, intense emotionality is associated not with weakness but with power. In Homer's *Odyssey*, for example, the protagonist, a paragon of forceful leadership, weeps copiously at several points when he loses beloved friends in battle. And yet the ancient Greeks clearly did not consider Odysseus a wimp.

Finally, I put more pressure on trainees with a paranoid streak than I do with others to keep giving me evaluations of my supervision and what they would want to change about our collaboration. Part of a paranoid orientation toward the world is a tendency to keep secrets, and a penchant toward secrecy is the enemy of clinical maturation. Because of their tendency to disown internal reactions and to project that mental content onto others, paranoid supervisees have a special need for opportunities to learn that honest feedback is not inevitably damaging to a relationship.

It is not easy for paranoid individuals to comply with directives to say what they feel. It takes time. It frightens them to be direct; they anticipate reprisals and can be extremely slow to assimilate the absence of payback for attitudes toward supervisors that are not somehow "correct." Despite all the challenges they present for supervision, I should add that even though it can be difficult to adapt to their psychology, I have found it gratifying to consult with clinicians whose personalities contain significant paranoia. These sensitive people suffer a lot, try hard to be good therapists, and have high ethical standards. They can flourish in the context of respect for those qualities.

Schizoid Dynamics in Supervision

Interestingly, the supervisors and consultants who have had the deepest and most lasting influence on me as a therapist have described themselves unapologetically as schizoid. Their self-concept was influenced by phenomenological descriptions like those of Guntrip (1969) or Seinfeld (1991), rather than by trait-based models of categorizing personality *disorders* such as those on which the DSM and ICD diagnostic criteria were based. Individuals with schizoid psychologies are frequently attracted to a psychoanalytic vocation. They are exquisitely sensitive to affect, enjoy thinking about foundational human questions, are intimately acquainted with parts of mental life that are unconscious for most of the rest of us (if one's primary defense is withdrawal, one has little need for distorting defenses), and are attracted to the ways that psychoanalytic practice can resolve their conflict about closeness versus distance (see Wheelis, 1956). Clinical engagement allows them a powerful experience of intimacy, but within the context of reliable boundaries of time, place, and role.

I feel a natural warmth toward schizoid people, and I greatly enjoy consulting with therapists with central schizoid dynamics. They tend to be good at both empathic immersion and boundary definition. What can trip them up occurs in working with clingy, self-dramatizing patients, such as those with histrionic and/or borderline dynamics. One of my early mentors, self-diagnosed as schizoid, used to tell me that he could not work with such clients because he experienced them as "dishonest." In other words, they used repression, displacement, reaction formation, acting out, and other defenses that were alien to his own psychology. He preferred working with psychotic patients because he felt that their suffering is "real."

The fact that some people are profoundly extroverted and relationship oriented can seem as weird to a schizoid person as the profound introversion of the schizoid person can seem to those of us who tend to see others as sources of comfort and pleasure (rather than of impingement and irritation). A supervisor's sensitivity to a schizoid personality tendency is particularly critical given that avoidant attachment styles, which can be assumed to be more common in schizoid people, have been empirically associated with worse supervisory outcomes (Mesrie, Diener, & Clark, 2018; Wrape, Callahan, Rieck, & Watkins, 2017).

Even though people with schizoid dynamics often worry about going crazy, and even though they feel a sense of kinship with people in states of psychosis, a schizoid psychology does not equate with pathology (see McWilliams, 2006, for the thinking behind this assertion). Supervision with a schizoid person will go better if the supervisee feels that his or her quirky, imaginative, artistic sensibility is appreciated without judgment. It will also benefit if the supervisor tries to help the schizoid clinician to mentalize the internal world of extroverted, needy, and sometimes theatrical individuals. If they can be patient with their defenses, schizoid therapists can be particularly healing to intensely reactive clients, who learn in the presence of a consistently nonreactive other that their own boundaries are safe from impingement and traumatic penetration.

If the mentor has a schizoid streak, the supervisee will know it intuitively—in fact, the supervisor may have been sought out initially because the student or junior colleague sensed in him or her the presence of a kindred spirit. The supervisory alliance can benefit greatly from the supervisor's acknowledgment of personal acquaintance with schizoid experience. The supervisee can feel warmly approached as a fellow member of a tribe of the solitary. The pairing of a schizoid supervisor and schizoid supervisee permits the trainee to see *in vivo* that even though schizoid dynamics may make social and personal life difficult, they can be quite valuable in clinical work.

Hysterical (Histrionic) Dynamics in Supervision

People with hysterical (histrionic) dynamics[1] are comparably sensitive, but their defenses against the feelings that threaten their equilibrium are different. Central to hysterical and histrionic dynamics are a vulnerability to overstimulation; a feeling of internal smallness or weakness; and a tendency to orient toward issues of gender, sexuality, and power. Individuals with such issues handle overstimulation by milder forms of denial and dissociation, by regression, and by displacement, sometimes creating distracting crises that they experience as "happening to" them

---

[1] I am using "hysterical" and "histrionic" to refer to points on a continuum of severity; the fact that the latter dynamic has historically been used to describe the more severe and unregulated versions of hysterical psychology is one reason the DSM labels the relevant personality *disorder* as histrionic.

rather than as reflecting any operation of their own agency. Because their cognitive style is impressionistic (Shapiro, 1965), they need their supervisors to ask for details and to investigate the particulars of clinical descriptions that sound vague or minimized.

Like individuals with depressive and masochistic tendencies, clinicians with hysterical dynamics usually present few obvious obstacles to supervision. Most of my comments about working with these therapists apply equally to more hysterically organized clinicians. Like depressive therapists, they want to please and may idealize in a pleasant way, and they need to be similarly encouraged toward critical thinking and an appreciation of the complexity of their internal reactions. They need to find their own power rather than feeling themselves always to be the victim of forces beyond their control. One of my psychiatrist colleagues is sometimes confronted with helpless appeals to her authority from histrionically inclined residents facing a difficult clinical situation that they will have to learn to handle. She will gently tease the therapist: "Yes, this patient needs a *doctor*. Oh yes, *you* are a doctor, aren't you? What response do you think is called for?"

When problems arise in mentoring individuals who are more hysterical, issues of gender, sexuality, and power are frequently central. In this territory, the most problematic supervisory dyad may be the combination of a female therapist with hysterical tendencies and a heterosexual male supervisor who has narcissistic needs to be seen as insightful and competent. The problem is that she needs to find her own insightfulness and competence, and he wants to show her his own. In the worst versions of this familiar story, the supervisor cannot contain his need to demonstrate his superiority, and the supervisee handles her sense of inferiority, or her sense that she is being *seen* as inferior, by a subtle seductiveness intended (often unconsciously) to recalibrate the balance of power between the parties in the supervisory dyad. The supervisor then feels distracted and/or sexually attracted, and the supervision may lose its proper focus. Similar power struggles are sometimes inferable in the converse dyad, in which a heterosexual male therapist with hysterical tendencies is in supervision with a narcissistically inclined heterosexual female supervisor. Related problems can also plague supervisees and supervisors with same-sex orientations if one or both have significant hysterical dynamics.

For any clinician mentoring someone with a hysterical psychology, an overriding concern should be to help the supervisee find an internal sense of agency, solidity, and maturity, even when faced with patients' intense affect or upsetting transferences. Rather than immediately offering one's own take on the supervisee's clinical material, it is important to get into the habit of asking what the therapist thinks is going on. Pressing for details is important. Inquiring into countertransference is valuable but should be done slowly and tentatively, as people with hysterical dynamics can easily feel penetrated and exposed.

It is also critical to take hysterically oriented supervisees seriously, even when their style is self-mocking or self-dramatizing. Doing so can be counterintuitive, because in the expectation of others' contempt for them, people with hysterical dynamics tend to preemptively provoke condescending responses (the "neurotic paradox" or "self-fulfilling prophecy"). They subtly make fun of themselves or dramatize affective states in ways that make these emotions come across as false. Supervisors have to remind themselves that the feelings are actually accurate; it is simply the presentation, suffused with anxieties about how their communications will be received, that makes the content feel phony. I am aware of how difficult it can be to take seriously a person who is self-dramatizing or seductive or comes across as a wide-eyed child, but supervisees who relate in these ways are particularly in need of respect for their capacities to be authentic, professional, and adult. Eventually, the cutesy gestures should fade out.

Even much astute psychoanalytic writing in this territory has not succeeded in avoiding a patronizing tone. Because individuals with hysterical tendencies are often treated dismissively, it is particularly important to relate to them with respect as competent grown-ups. It is hard for a supervisee to take in the *content* of a supervisor's teaching when the *process* includes overtones of disdain. I know this from personal experience, and I am grateful to my analytic supervisors for insisting on taking me seriously even when I was trying to get by on charm, at a time when sexist assumptions about male normativity dominated both psychoanalysis and American society.

Obsessive–Compulsive Dynamics in Supervision

In sharp contrast to supervisees with more hysterical tendencies, those with obsessive and compulsive psychologies are anything but impressionistic. Their problem is that they notice every tree and miss the forest. Rather than feeling overwhelmed by emotions that they must then minimize, they may have no access to most of their affective life, which they handle by intellectual defenses and compartmentalization. They approach supervision with the wish to master an approach at a cognitive level, and they may seem to view the complexities of clinical work as somehow a mess that they need a formula to clean up. The combination of an obsessive supervisor with an obsessive supervisee can lead to very interesting academic conversations that fail to foster the emotional maturation characteristic of supervision at its best.

The mistakes that obsessional therapists make typically result from approaching clinical work cerebrally. For example, a male therapist I recently consulted with told me about a prospective client who stated that his reason for coming was that he wanted to figure out if his girlfriend was borderline. The therapist was intrigued with this question, accepted the premise, and spent the session talking with the client about the DSM criteria for diagnosing borderline personality disorder, eventually deciding with him that she indeed met those specifications. The client left the meeting in what the therapist described as a good mood, apparently feeling supported in his conviction that the problems in his relationship were all a result of his girlfriend's personality pathology. My colleague was surprised that the man did not return. But he had completely neglected to find out what the client's own story was or to consider the feelings and defenses behind his need to pathologize his girlfriend. In retrospect, the therapist could see his own failing, but at the time, he had become intellectually engrossed in ways that led to his compromising his therapeutic role.

Obsessional clinicians work hard to do the right thing, and for this reason it is easy to admire them and enjoy their earnest intelligence. But it is part of a supervisor's job to loosen them up for their own sakes and for the potential benefit to their patients. The downside of the obsessive style includes a grim seriousness; overthinking; and the inability to enjoy playfulness, access imagination, value intuitive leaps, or call on humor to transform clinical tedium. When one is supervising therapists who have tendencies to isolate affect, intellectualize, rationalize, and compartmentalize, one usually has to confront them pretty hard about their evasions of affect. Simply observing their avoidance of feeling can lead to an intellectual acknowledgment without emotional insight.

Obsessional supervisees are overconcerned with what is correct versus incorrect technique. Teasing, telling jokes, and sharing amusing stories may help in the process of undermining an excessively obsessional approach to clinical work and expanding a space for play (Winnicott, 1971). Role play may help to enliven rule-bound clinicians; by having to "become" the patient, they can engage in physical imitation that may connect them to affect. Supervisors can challenge the binary notions of correct versus incorrect, helping them to expand into the realm of the creative and spontaneous and to enjoy the playful and pleasurable aspects of being a therapist.

Posttraumatic Dynamics in Supervision

It is no secret that many of us chose to become therapists because we were trying to understand and master a traumatic history. Personal trauma can lay the groundwork for empathy, patience, and other clinically essential attitudes. But such a background does present challenges. Those of us who bear witness to the traumatic accounts of our patients may be easily triggered emotionally, especially if a patient's experiences resemble traumatic incidents in our past. The dangers of secondary or vicarious traumatization have been well documented (Gartner, 2014; Pearlman & Saakvitne, 1995; Walker, 2004); they apply to all clinicians but especially to those of us with histories of abuse, neglect, bullying, rape, combat, and other traumatizing experiences.

Therapists struggling with posttraumatic issues can be greatly helped by supervisors who ask matter-of-factly about whether they have undergone personal trauma, who are open to their talking about what the patient's account evokes in them, and who help them with self-care and strategies to prevent or reduce secondary traumatization (see Walker, 2004). It is useful to acknowledge their reactivity and normalize it, as most trauma survivors have a running internal conversation characterized by self-attack (for "overreacting," being "too fragile," for not being "professional" enough, for thinking they could be a therapist in the first place, and so on). If the supervisor has a trauma history and is comfortable saying so (in a casual tone suggesting that such experiences are simply facts of life that therapists have to take into account), such a disclosure may help supervisees to deal realistically with their own posttraumatic vulnerability.

Patients with histories of trauma can be unusually sensitive to the mental states of others. It is not uncommon for them to notice therapists' countertransferences to their devastating stories. When clients pick up their distress or dissociation in session, supervisees may need advice about how to respond. It can be a great relief to them to learn that is not against any rules to say to their patients something like, "I do want you to talk about all this, but it is difficult to hear what you've been through, and you're right that I was starting to space out. Thanks for pulling me back into connection." The fact that one can simply admit the difficulty of staying present when trauma invades the interpersonal space may allow the supervisee's patients to be less self-critical toward their own lapses into states of disconnection and trance.

Finally, therapists with traumatic pasts may need supervisory help in identifying clinical populations that may overwhelm their adaptive capacities. It is not uncommon for people to go into this field hoping to help those who have suffered the same way they did—and then realize that they cannot bear that work. A mentor can reasonably suggest that early-career therapists with this problem avoid having too many traumatized patients or specializing with posttraumatic groups. They may not know yet that there is no shame in being realistic about which kinds of clients one does and does not do well with, respectively. Once their basic education in psychotherapy is completed and they are credentialed, they will have considerable leeway in choosing their professional focus, and they should do so with some attention to self-care.

Narcissistic Dynamics in Supervision

My own greatest supervisory challenges have involved working with supervisees who struck me as significantly narcissistic. Their preoccupations with self-image went beyond ordinary discomfort with being observed and evaluated; they had to be right, could not receive constructive criticism without feeling attacked, looked down on others, and viewed training as a competition to be seen as "the best." They may not have met DSM criteria for narcissistic personality disorder, but their mental life seemed dominated by concerns with status, power, wealth, and attractiveness. I am conceptualizing them as located on the lower tiers of Kernberg's (e.g., 2014a) narcissistic continuum, which runs from normal narcissistic concerns at the top, through neurotic narcissism, narcissistic personality disorder, malignant narcissism, and outright psychopathy (antisocial personality).

I would guess that in North American communities in this era, when psychoanalytic training is no longer a ticket to wealth and high status, most analytically oriented programs have only a small number of trainees whose personalities are dominated by narcissistic dynamics; most contemporary students of psychoanalysis choose the profession because of an attraction to its subject matter rather than for prestige. This was not the case when the field had more social cachet. Readers of a certain age may recall a number of analysts who behaved arrogantly enough, especially to nonanalysts, to give psychoanalysis a bad name. Currently, some notably narcissistic students might be found in highly ranked graduate programs, markedly competitive internships and residencies, and prominent institutes, to which they are attracted because of their prestige, but they seem to be uncommon outside those bastions of psychoanalytic status.

I have worked with a few supervisees who seemed to me fundamentally narcissistic. Some have functioned rather well in the role of therapist. I have had colleagues whose self-enhancing agendas seem clear but who also seem to have a good track record with patients. People with the central narcissistic dynamics of idealization and devaluation can be quite perceptive, especially of others' self-esteem issues, and they are often bright and knowledgeable. But unless a narcissistic supervisee stays in a prolonged state of idealization and the supervisor's self-regard thrives on being idealized, working with a narcissistic trainee can be painful.

The main problem for supervisors is that people who expect themselves to know everything already find it hard to acknowledge the need to take anything in. These sensitive yet extremely defensive people, who are so invested in protecting an impossibly flawless persona (the grandiose self), frequently cannot bear hearing that their clinical work could be improved. My experience is that all goes well in supervision as long as I am unfailingly supportive and validating. But eventually, inevitably, I feel the therapist has made a mistake or could profit from thinking differently about a clinical issue. As soon as I enter that territory, the supervisee devalues my input and finds ways to ascribe it to my personal or professional failings.

I once worked with a graduate student who was quite performative in her style of case presentation. In her supervision group, she would participate with an attitude of "I can show you how it's done" rather than "I could use your help." In one of her case presentations that involved a young boy in play therapy, her classmates and I had some ideas for deepening the treatment. When I offered one such suggestion, she bristled and suggested that I was ignorant of recent developments in child psychoanalysis. Each time she got critical feedback, she seemed hurt and offended that she had not simply been admired. Her argumentativeness tended to irritate both me and her fellow students. Correctly identifying our annoyance, she concluded that we were looking for a scapegoat. In a state of self-righteous anger, she announced that she was leaving the group because she could not work with a professor who fostered such destructive dynamics.

As in this instance, I have found that when I supervise or consult with colleagues who have significant narcissism, I often find myself in a distinctive dilemma. Their defense against their pain at being seen as imperfect quickly becomes a narrative about my own psychopathology, one that explains my purported insensitivity and misunderstanding. I recall one very bright and talented man, for example, to whom I had mentioned in some relevant context (during a honeymoon period in our early work) that my father had been intimidating. When I switched from undiluted support of his clinical skill to suggesting he could have done something differently, he said it was clear from my comments that I had a problem with men and was acting out a negative father transference toward him.

In such situations of implicit or explicit fault finding by a person trying to protect narcissistic defenses, I typically feel in a bind. I could say something like, "I don't think it's a father transference; I think I simply had a difference of opinion with you about the best way to help the client." Alternatively, I could say, "There certainly may be elements of a father transference in my relationship to you, but even if that's true, I think it would be valuable for you to look at the content of what I said about your approach to the patient." If I choose to respond in the first way, I usually get written off as defensive. If I respond in the second way, the supervisee typically hears only the first clause of my sentence and files the rest mentally as "She admitted that it's her problem, not mine, so I don't have to think about this anymore." In other words, I find myself trapped in a paranoid–schizoid, doer–done-to, binary stalemate.

I have not yet found a good way to create or restore a sense of the supervisory alliance when an impasse like this happens. Sometimes one can get some traction by asking a genuinely inquisitive question along the lines of, "How would you go about discerning the difference between my mistake due to my blindness to my dynamics and your mistake due to yours?" Eventually, the supervisor might have to say something like, "I guess we've come to a point when you have to decide whether there's anything more you can learn from me," and see whether the supervisee is capable of acknowledging any ongoing need for the supervisory relationship.

For analytic clinicians, it is natural to address impasses by talking in these kinds of ways about the pattern itself rather than engaging on one side of a binary. Unfortunately, with narcissistic supervisees such attempts tend to recreate the dilemma because the trainee feels even more attacked and gets even more defensive, as if having *any* dynamics or participating in *any* enactments compels a verdict of inadequacy. Parenthetically, the example of the assumed father transference speaks to the potential risks of self-disclosures with narcissistic mentees: They may become fuel for the person's defensive avoidance of real connection.

Most mentors learn to be careful about personal disclosures to narcissistic supervisees, just as we are with narcissistic patients, who may devalue us instantly if we suddenly seem ordinary and human and not the paragons constructed by their idealizing imaginations.

It is a shame that we face this complication, as it could be therapeutic for narcissistic supervisees, just as it is for patients with pathological narcissism, for us to exemplify a stance of acknowledging ordinary failings and blind spots with no loss to our self-esteem. For those whose subjectivity is dominated by narcissism, if one is not perfect or omnipotent or a "winner," one is a failure, a chump, a "loser." If we could help them out of this polarity, we would be doing both ourselves and them a great service, potentially improving not only their clinical relationships but also their personal attachments.

I do not have a wealth of ideas about how to transform work with a narcissistically defended supervisee into the steadily more emotionally honest, searching collaboration that it can become with individuals who have other core dynamics. It helps considerably if they have had enough therapy to be aware of their psychology, but that takes time, as they typically approach their own treatment as an opportunity to complain about others. But I have a consoling thought: Narcissistic people do learn. Unfortunately for our own narcissistic needs as supervisors, they do not give us the satisfaction of acknowledging that they learned something *from us*. Instead, they absorb our ideas and claim them later as theirs. If our own narcissism is sufficiently tamed, the fact that they improve clinically in response to supervision is a kind of comfort, albeit cold.

Psychopathic Dynamics in Supervision

Very occasionally, one encounters a supervisee who seems to be at the psychopathic end of the narcissistic spectrum. Such individuals may cheat, flatter, seduce, and manipulate their way through training programs. They have a remarkable talent for ingratiating themselves with people in positions of power and slipping under the radar of systems designed to identify lapses in ethical functioning. With supervisors, they master the persona of the earnest, devoted student of therapy, and because they can be extremely good at portraying that character, it can be impossible to see their dissimulation for what it is. Fortunately, their peers are seldom blind to their maneuvers. Hence, supervision groups and other opportunities for a supervisor to observe how they behave with people who do not have something they want can be valuable in identifying and modifying their power-oriented motives.

First, I should say that individuals whose mental life is dominated by psychopathy should not be therapists. They will throw under the bus anyone who interferes with their own agenda, including patients, colleagues, and mentors. They have no use for honesty, the fundamental value behind psychoanalytic exploration. Their version of "empathy" involves a remarkable capacity to perceive the vulnerabilities of others without any care for their welfare. Given their skill in managing appearances, ingenuity at exploiting the trust of others (including supervisors), and penchant for disappearing and resurfacing elsewhere when their machinations are exposed, it is difficult to remove them from the field if they are determined to occupy a clinical role.

I know of a few instances in which a clearly psychopathic person who was denied graduation from a training program or had a license revoked after committing unethical acts found another route to being a clinician and eventually went into practice. Individuals with psychopathy can be dangerously litigious, a tendency that makes faculty members think twice about expelling them. And they usually have on their side at least one kindhearted authority whom they have persuaded to believe they have been gravely misunderstood. But we should nevertheless attempt to prevent them from occupying legitimate practice roles by sharing our concerns with colleagues and maintaining appropriate paper trails.

That said, there are some people who behave psychopathically only in certain situations, either because of distrust of particular authorities, or because they have been encouraged to cheat in the service of specific goals, or because Machiavellian strategies have worked for them and have never been challenged. These individuals are not thoroughly antisocial, and if their core values are compatible with clinical service, they can be influenced to be better versions of themselves. The best corrective to a manipulative pattern is suffering consequences that cannot be finessed by connivance and charm. Clinicians with a psychopathic streak tend to give short shrift to paperwork and similar administrative obligations, and so it is important for supervisors of therapists suspected of antisocial tendencies to keep an eye on their record-keeping and other more bureaucratic and boring aspects of professional practice. Small, less visible details of the supervisee's functioning should be checked on periodically.

It is critical not to relax the regular rules and procedures for students with possible psychopathy. I have rarely supervised antisocial clinicians, but I have treated some therapists who were their classmates and have heard numerous stories of special deals that a calculating student was able to pull off by taking advantage of a soft-hearted authority in a training program. Although making thoughtful exceptions to general policies can be appropriate for individuals without a tendency toward manipulation, giving special breaks to students with psychopathic traits reinforces their sense of entitlement and their habit of "working the system" rather than learning how to function with integrity. Finally, in instances when their machinations get them into trouble, supervisors should not rescue them from the consequences of their own behavior.

OTHER ASPECTS OF INDIVIDUALITY: IMPLICATIONS FOR SUPERVISION

In addition to diagnostic conceptualizations, there are many other aspects of individuality that may affect the supervisory relationship and have implications for the alliance. Supervisor and supervisee have their respective temperaments, sexual and gender orientations and identities, ethnic and racial influences and identifications, spiritual or religious backgrounds and interests, and political perspectives and commitments. In addition, either person might be, for example, an adoptee, a twin or triplet, a "replacement child" for a dead sibling, a cancer survivor, or a person with a chronic illness or physical limitation. The supervisor and/ or supervisee may have a history of addiction, an eating disorder, or bipolar illness or psychosis. All such factors can contribute to a personal disposition that includes both blind spots and special perceptiveness.

I am not a fan of conceptualizing the supervisor's adaptation to such differences as "competencies," as this locution implies that one can eventually master what one needs to know about an infinite range of experiences of diversity. It is simply not possible to be "competent" with respect to all of the important potential differences between supervisor and supervisee. But perhaps most relevant to my own attitude is Fors's (2018, p. 82) argument that "from a psychoanalytic standpoint, the worst theoretical problem with the concept of cultural competency is the underlying assumption that prejudice is something that can remit completely on the basis of cognitive education."

As I noted in the Introduction, some scholars have defined overall supervisory competency or learning objectives in ways that do not preclude nuanced relational work (e.g., Killingmo et al., 2014; Moga & Cabaniss, 2014; Strømme, 2012; Watkins, 2013b, 2016). Such definitions have the advantage of being operationalized for research purposes; they permit the measurement and statistical manipulation of values at a time when more research into the supervisory process is sorely needed. But I think that adapting the model of attaining various "competencies" to the area of diversity stretches the skills-training metaphor beyond its useful limits, as it does not always translate into sensitive adaptation to supervisees who bring unique minority perspectives to clinical work, and it does not sufficiently appreciate the internalized and unconscious prejudices of the therapist.

It is reasonable to expect mentors to be knowledgeable about some implications of general categories of differences (e.g., race, gender, sexuality, ethnicity, and traumatic histories of certain groups), but specific knowledge (e.g., about how racism, sexism, heterosexism, cultural prejudice, or a great-grandparent's traumatic past has affected a particular supervisee) cannot be realistically expected of any supervisor in the absence of a conversation. For practitioners, just as the research-based criterion of symptom reduction fails to capture the "vital signs" (see Chapter 3) indicating clinically significant progress in therapy, the concepts defined for research purposes do not always capture what is most germane to good mentorship—especially in the realm of individual uniqueness.

In recent decades, there has been an explosion of psychoanalytic literature about race (e.g., Akhtar, 2014; Davids, 2011; Holmes, 1992, 2016; Leary, 2000; Suchet, 2007); gender (e.g., Corbett, 2011; Ehrensaft, 2014; Harris, 2008; Lemma, 2018); sexuality (e.g., Abrevaya & Thomson-Salo, 2019; Dimen, 2014; Drescher, 2015); able-bodiedness (Davis, 1995; McRuer, 2006; Solomon, 2012); culture (e.g., Gherovici & Christian, 2018; Tummala-Narra, 2016); class and social privilege (e.g., Ainslie, 2011; Fors, 2018; Layton, Hollander, & Gutwill, 2006; Ryan, 2018); colonialism and political oppression (e.g., Greedharry, 2008; Layton & Leavy-Sperounis, 2020); and the intergenerational transmission of trauma (e.g., Brothers, 2014; Grand & Salberg, 2017; Kim & Strathearn, 2017). There have also been numerous efforts to theorize about difference at a "meta" level (e.g., Fors, 2018; Gentile, 2018; Saketopoulou, 2011; Young-Bruehl, 2007). This intersectional work has been a welcome corrective in a field appropriately criticized for its historically white, Western European, patriarchal, heterosexist monoculture.

Adequate theoretical and empirical literature on diversity that focuses explicitly on supervision, especially psychoanalytic supervision, is only beginning to emerge (e.g., Brown, 2010; Foster, Moskowitz, & Javier, 1996; Harrell, 2014; Hawkins & Shohet, 2012; Inman & DeBoer Kreider, 2013; Pieterse, 2018; Power, 2009; Schen & Greenlee, 2018; Tummala-Narra, 2004, 2009; Watkins & Hook, 2016; Watkins et al.,

2019; Watson, Raju, & Soklaridis, 2017). There is even less scholarship that explores supervisory dyads in which the supervisor occupies a less socially privileged position than the supervisee. I have always considered myself fairly sensitive to diversity issues, but in the second edition of the *Psychodynamic Diagnostic Manual* (Lingiardi & McWilliams, 2017), I failed to notice that all the examples we gave pertaining to matters of marginality and difference assumed a therapist in the dominant group and a patient in a subordinate one (see Drescher & Fors, 2018). As in the case of so many phenomena that cause discomfort when exposed, I was looking at the data through the unconscious lenses of privilege.

Because empathy and attunement are not powerful enough alone to counteract ignorance, it is important for supervisors to have some acquaintance with the literature on race, gender, and sexuality. But we also need a willingness to learn from our supervisees about such issues *as they pertain to them individually.* This task is not always easy. Supervisees in social minorities often report fatigue from having to raise the consciousness of yet another person about common experiences of those in their group. Many people of color in the United States, for example, are currently finding that the emotional burden of educating white clinicians about racism has become exhausting. They are weary of the role of racial sensitizer. Nevertheless, I have noted that when supervisees have concluded that I am genuinely interested in learning from them, those who are significantly different from me have been gracious about educating me about the nuances of their own situation and grateful that I am not applying some boilerplate set of assumptions to their experience.

Equally key to progress in supervision are supervisors' efforts to acknowledge and explore their own dark sides nondefensively. Such openness may potentiate the same moral courage in supervisees. Inevitably, certain prejudices will accompany anyone's location in various social hierarchies, and although admitting to them is painful, it can foster the habit of honesty that is central to the psychoanalytic ethos. In a paper unusual for the frankness of its self-disclosure, Anne Power (2009) wrote:

> When supervision works well it enables us to access and think about our most difficult countertransference; this will sometimes include oppressive and hostile feelings towards vulnerable minorities. Supervisors are familiar with facilitating and containing difficult affects but in my experience as supervisee and supervisor I find difference is, not surprisingly perhaps, the hardest place to go. (p. 158)

One of the frequent complaints of clinicians with minority identifications is that psychoanalysts tend to use the hammer of traditional analytic theories to make everything they fail to understand into a nail that they can pound with that hammer. In a survey of Italian psychoanalysts, Lingiardi and Capozzi (2004) found that despite conscious adherence to less pathologizing paradigms, many of them still depended on developmental models that pathologize homosexual variants of maturation. Drescher's (2002) account of his psychoanalytic training is replete with instances of his mentors' misunderstandings and efforts to graft his own experiences onto heteronormativity. Analysts who identify as sexually straight may find the territory of heterosexual oedipal dynamics familiar and safe, and hence tend to apply such metaphors to all clinical material, regardless of a patient's sexual orientation. In contrast, empathy with being gay requires a leap of imagination for a heterosexual therapist. Many of us currently show a similar resistance to identification with trans experiences.

Similarly, in the film *Black Psychoanalysts Speak* (Winograd, 2014), analysts of color have described how their teachers and supervisors avoided discussing the traumatic effects of racism and instead framed their own and their minority patients' experiences of mistreatment in terms of ordinary developmental challenges. Despite the efforts that psychoanalytic institutes are currently making to increase attention to issues of diversity, the assumption persists, with some evidence to support it, that psychoanalytic education is ignorant of or indifferent to diversity. In a recent account of an in-process survey for the American Psychoanalytic Association, Hart and colleagues (2020) identified a significant number of potential candidates for analytic training who believe that institutes adhere to monocultural norms that they view as "standard procedure," have a tokenistic approach to diversity issues, operate as if sufficient empathy makes the study of sociocultural identities unnecessary, or give inadequate attention to the exclusionary history of psychoanalysis. Supervisors need to be sensitive to this perception and take pains to address it with honesty about the elements in the stereotype that have a basis in fact.

In recent surveys of supervisees of mentors of varying theoretical orientations, the question of the supervisor's sensitivity to difference has loomed large. Gregus, Stevens, Seivert, Tucker, and Callahan (2020) found that mentees from underrepresented groups were considerably more likely to complain of their supervisor's insensitivity to diversity issues or lack of knowledge of the literature on cultural competence (see Hawkins & Shohet, 2012; Watkins & Hook, 2016; Watkins et al.,

2019). Research on supervisee self-disclosure shows that it is students in minority groups who are most reluctant to open up to mentors about diversity issues, often because when they have tried, they have encountered defensiveness (Callahan & Love, 2020).

CONCLUDING COMMENTS

I have tried in this chapter to bring some specific angles of vision to the challenge of adapting to the particular psychologies of individual supervisees, taking into account the supervisor's own dynamics. I have shared some ideas about supervisory problems and solutions that arise in the context of several personality dynamics, including depressive and masochistic, paranoid, schizoid, hysterical, obsessive–compulsive, post-traumatic, narcissistic, and psychopathic psychologies. I have tried to scratch the surface of some supervisory issues as they relate to areas of diversity, including gender, sexuality, race and ethnicity, ability, class, culture, religious and spiritual background and affinities, political orientation, oppression, and other instances of uniqueness and marginality in both supervisor and supervisee. Overall, I have put the greatest emphasis on a combination of openness to being taught and acknowledgment of one's own areas of privilege, prejudice, and ignorance. I hope the reader is left with the take-home message of the value of both knowledge and humility in the supervisory encounter.

Chapter Nine

■ ■ ■ ■

Getting the Most Out of Supervision

FOR SUPERVISEES

This chapter is directed toward readers who are currently in either required or voluntary supervision, whether they are beginners in graduate programs in counseling and psychotherapy or seasoned clinicians in advanced psychoanalytic training. It will probably be most relevant to relatively new supervisees and those for whom supervised hours are mandatory. It may be helpful as well to their mentors and perhaps to students in courses on supervision. In Chapter 3 of *Psychoanalytic Psychotherapy* (McWilliams, 2004), I made some observations about the optimal use of supervision. Having heard from students that those ideas were useful to them, I try here to treat more extensively the question of how to maximize what can be learned from one's supervisory experiences.

OVERALL BENEFITS AND GOALS OF PSYCHOANALYTIC SUPERVISION

In addition to helping you in practical ways with your clinical understanding and skills, psychoanalytic supervision should support your growth as a self-directed professional. It should help you acknowledge without defensiveness any areas of difficulty you find yourself having with clients, especially those that seem to recur in your work, and yet at the same time it should increase your feelings of confidence as a practitioner. It should build on your natural intuition and compassion, helping you integrate those qualities comfortably into how you behave in the role of therapist. It should give you a sense of safety about self-disclosure that will transfer to an ability to put your patients at ease when they confess painful and shame-ridden parts of their inner world. It should even provide space for playfulness (Aronson, 2000). It should offer opportunities for identification that eventually result in an internal template for your self-supervision going forward and for your own future work as a supervisor.

Clinical work is both emotionally and cognitively demanding. In the affective realm, patients can bring out aspects of ourselves that surprise and even shock us (e.g., sadistic fantasies, trance states, boredom, feelings of humiliation). It is hard to get used to the emotional demands of doing psychotherapy; most graduate programs—especially those led by academics without much ongoing clinical experience—do not prepare you for how emotionally exhausting practice can be (see Boyd-Franklin et al., 2015). As someone who is both an academic and a therapist, I can attest confidently that there is nothing in the role of teaching, research, or general scholarship that even remotely resembles absorbing the intensely painful, intimate affects of one suffering person for 45 or 50 minutes.

In the cognitive realm, it can be difficult to take in the fact that even when a particular approach has shown its superiority based on statistical averages, the person in front of you is not a statistical average. That individual requires an adaptation to his or her particular psychology. And even when therapy is done sensitively, most clinical choices do not involve a right versus a wrong way to help a unique client. Sometimes, clinical choices are not even questions of better and worse. They tend to be trade-offs, with both positive and negative aspects to each possible solution to a clinical problem. Efforts to connect therapeutically involve complex combinations of listening and talking by a specific therapist at a specific time to a specific person. This is the artistic aspect of clinical work.

As with any skill, general competence in psychotherapy is a lifelong project. It may be hard to approach supervision with the mental set that everything you do can probably be improved, but the sooner you get used to the experience of learning an art (as opposed to carrying out an objectively measurable task in dutiful accordance with some prescription), the better. To complicate matters, learning to think and speak in psychoanalytic jargon can be daunting. It can take a couple of years to master the idiosyncratic concepts pervading psychoanalytic literature, which tend to be rooted in metaphors that shift and evolve, as the images that capture clinicians' lived experiences change over time. To complicate matters, the same term may mean something slightly different to different supervisors.

Successive generations of theory constructors have enjoyed contributing new concepts and metaphors that capture particular psychological processes. This need to offer something fresh not only makes it difficult to research psychoanalytic ideas (Westen, 2002), but it also makes it hard for newcomers to engage with a tradition of thinking that contains more than a century of evolving metaphors, from Freud's expropriation of the language and images of physics ("cathexis," "sublimation") to our current efforts to express attachment processes ("inner working model," "safe harbor"). You may not be accustomed to talking in peculiar locutions such as "object relations," "superego lacunae," "the paranoid–schizoid position," "the repetition compulsion," "narcissistic extension," "the unthought known," "transitional space," or "the third." But if you are a caring person, you already have the basic equipment for being an effective psychodynamic clinician. Good supervisors will appreciate and build on that foundation, helping you amalgamate your natural human relations skills with this strange, slippery professional language.

The ultimate consequence of effective psychoanalytic supervision involves the integration of two maturational accomplishments: (1) the assimilation of enough helpful direction from your mentors that you can eventually rely on a calm, benevolent, and reliable "internal supervisor" (Casement, 1985), who helps you respond to your clients in ways that are natural and spontaneous as well as inherently therapeutic, and (2) the evolution of a clear sense of when you should seek consultation, even after you have successfully cleared all the hurdles that may currently lie between you and professional legitimacy or autonomy. Let me elaborate on each of these supervisory outcomes.

Developing a Reliable Internal Supervisor

Internalizing a supportive supervisory "voice" requires that you do your part to make each experience of supervision as useful as possible to your current work and future growth. Even if you are stuck with a mentor for whom you have very little respect, it is up to you to find something you can learn from that person (if only how *not* to act with your future supervisees). The worst enemy of learning is getting fixed in the posture of complaining about what *should be* rather than making the best adaptation to what *is*.

This may not be easy. I have noticed in recent years that agency sites emphasize and support supervision considerably less than they once did. Hospitals and counseling centers are currently under relentless pressure to "do more with less"—a maddeningly patronizing piece of self-serving magical thinking that invites clinicians to spin straw into gold. Whereas in a previous era most mentors would have had the time and institutional backing to help you become a better therapist, they may now have to supervise you almost on the run. In the face of current systemic stresses, they may have to spend the scant time they have available educating you about risk-management issues and required record-keeping rather than getting into the weeds of clinical topics.

Recent interns and trainees consistently tell me that they feel they thrown into the deep end of the professional pool without a life jacket. They also get frequent implicit messages that the most vital concern of administrators is not the care of each patient but the protection and survival of the agency (cf. Menzies, 1960). This problem will probably not be responsive to complaints; its only solution is political action to get better funding for mental health. If you are being asked to treat difficult problems without adequate supervision, your job is simply to survive as well as you can and be honest with your clients about the limits of the services they receive. You can also keep reading, as much as it is possible to do so without exhausting yourself, because published articles and books on psychotherapy tend to be relatively uncontaminated by administrative issues.

Once you are more experienced and/or in a setting where supervisors have more time and resources to devote to your professional growth, you can probably negotiate with each mentor about how to work optimally together. Good supervisors and consultants typically invite such negotiation. By the time you approach graduation from your training program, you should know how you learn best and how to help your supervisor understand what ways of working are most helpful to you (for example, some of the clinicians I consult with are eager to role-play with me, while others feel awkward and distracted in doing so; some want to talk about one patient in great depth, while others prefer to present a different case each week). In the early years of your career, however, you will probably have to adapt to the way your supervisor wants to work and sometimes also to the ways prescribed by the organization with which he or she is affiliated.

Some supervisors will ask you to show a videotape of your session; others will want you to summarize it and then raise any concerns you have about your own interventions, the patient's psychology, or the transference–countertransference atmosphere. Some will want detailed process notes, while others will ask you instead for a more impressionistic overview. Some will expect you to have developed your own psychodynamic formulation; others prefer to do so collaboratively with you once they have the clinical data that you present. For reasons due to their individual personalities, theoretical predilections, and familiar patient populations, therapists differ greatly on how they prefer to supervise. Just as you are going through the process of finding which ways of working clinically are best suited to your own individuality, they have probably acquired some understanding of how they work best as supervisors.

For example, my husband does psychotherapy mostly with psychotic patients and supervises clinicians who want to improve their skills with this group. Before their supervisory meeting, he typically asks his supervisees to provide him an account of the session he will consult on that is as close to a transcript as they can recreate. Because making sense of psychotic communications requires close examination of the patient's words, and because the context is critical to decoding the patient's metaphorical ways of speaking, he wants the details. He likes to read the description the night before he consults with the therapist, so that he has time to develop a formulation that makes sense of what is outwardly quite confusing. Because a printed account of a session allows him to look back and forth at what came before and after each clinical interaction, he prefers the written record to a video.

For example, he recently described how a psychiatrist in training was taken aback when, seemingly out of the blue, a patient with psychotic symptoms demanded to know if he believed her claim that people were intruding into her apartment. Examination of the transcript showed that shortly before this demand, the patient had answered in the affirmative when the doctor had asked a routine history-taking question about whether she had ever been sexually abused. She had added that no one in her family had believed her at the time. Although it became apparent in supervision that there was a connection between the intrusion into her body during the childhood molestation and the current (delusional) intrusion into her apartment, and also between her early need for others to recognize a traumatic experience and her insistence on validation now, the clinician had not noticed the link because he was so startled by her sudden confrontation.

In contrast to this method of supervision, I have a strong preference *not* to have session descriptions transcribed and provided ahead of the scheduled supervisory hour. I am more of an auditory learner than my husband, who is more visual; hearing the material as the therapist conveys it helps me to observe my own immediate countertransference reactions and internal images. Because I work with mostly nonpsychotic patients, there is less material I need to decode and more material I need to understand in the context of the overall feeling tone of the work. When I am consulting with a therapist in the presence of other clinicians, my reporting on my ongoing internal process allows the audience to witness *in vivo* how I go about formulating a case. In such situations, there is thus an educational value to my operating in more unrehearsed ways.

For me, getting a transcript of the process ahead of time would miss some of the nuances. I want to hear how the therapist talks spontaneously about the patient. What feelings come through? What images are coming up in my mind? What experiences are suddenly alive in my memory? What song is going through my head? Why might those associations be getting triggered? How am I feeling toward the person presenting the case (i.e., what is the parallel process)? I like video recordings as well. When it is possible to do so, I get considerable help from watching a filmed session, especially of an initial meeting, which I used to do regularly when teaching a Rutgers course on psychodynamic interviewing. As I watched the clinical interaction unfold, I would ask myself these kinds of questions and share my internal process with class members.

Accommodating to a mentor's preferences may stretch you, including in some good ways. Ideally, your supervisor should be able to explain why he or she prefers a particular method of teaching. Try to cooperate even when you are asked to do something difficult. Although it can be burdensome, for example, to take extensive process notes, the discipline of that habit can contribute to a professional lifetime of noticing relevant clinical details. Whatever the approach of your supervisor, if you can identify with the rationale behind it (even if the approach itself leaves you cold), you will be constructing an internal presence that oversees a self-evaluating, self-supporting process that can be ongoing during your career.

Sometimes a supervisor will be strongly invested in proving the superiority of a particular psychoanalytic approach, such as ego psychology, object relations theory, self psychology, interpersonal or relational psychoanalysis, modern (Spotnitz-influenced) psychoanalysis, control–mastery theory, or Freudian, Jungian, Kleinian, or Lacanian theory. Sometimes the mentor will be a proponent of one of the procedures designed for a particular population, such as transference-focused psychotherapy or mentalization-based therapy for borderline psychologies, or one of the short-term models, such as accelerated experiential dynamic psychotherapy or intensive short-term dynamic psychotherapy. In these circumstances, it may be best to accept the supervisor's need to demonstrate the superiority of the preferred orientation and enjoy the benefits of learning from a partisan. If the supervisor enjoys comparing and contrasting approaches, you may be able to have stimulating conversations about clinical options, but if he or she is defensive and dogmatic, it will probably not facilitate the supervision for you to challenge the party line.

In such situations, you need to take what is positive and differentiate yourself later from what does not suit you and your clients. As I have noted, psychotherapy technique should be flexible, adaptable, and patient centered, not rigidly prescriptive. Any clinical intervention should be evaluated according to whether it moves the therapy forward—that is, whether the patient speaks with increasing freedom and shows progress in the vital signs of psychological wellness discussed in Chapter 3—rather than according to how well it approximates some idealized model of psychodynamic intervention. In other words, it should be judged by its effects, not its theoretical purity. Analysts who make contemptuous attacks on manualized cognitive-behavioral treatments easily forget the era when many psychodynamic therapists emerged from their training with an internal "orthodox committee" that critiqued them for every deviation from what was at the time considered correct analytic technique, irrespective of whether or not it helped the patient.

Knowing When to Go for Help

I have talked a lot in this book about the importance of overcoming the perfectionism from which many therapists suffer. At the same time that you need to be realistic and not perfectionistic about what can be achieved in treatment, you need also to make judgments about when your work feels inadequate, when you may be enacting something detrimental to the patient, or when you fall short of your own reasonable professional expectations. There are two areas in which I urge you to consider seeking consultation, no matter what stage of your career you

are in. The first involves areas in which any therapist would be advised
to get help; the second involves knowing when you are in risky territory
for idiosyncratic personal reasons.

In the first category are situations involving the relationship
between your work as a therapist and the larger society in which that
work goes on. They include challenges such as learning information
that you may have to report to public authorities, being asked by a
client for some kind of formal advocacy (e.g., a letter on a patient's
behalf), being asked for information by attorneys or other third parties,
being expected to give a deposition or court testimony about a patient,
receiving a subpoena for records, being notified of a complaint made
against you to a professional board, and so on. No matter how long you
have practiced, such situations should activate your internal supervisor's
immediate advice to hit the pause button and get direction from others
before taking any action.

In other words, learn how to stall. If it is a patient who asks for
some potentially problematic favor, you can always say, "Let me think
about what you're asking. I need time to reflect on how I feel about
that and about the possible unintended consequences of what you are
requesting." If the request is made by an attorney, you can say that you
are not able to respond immediately but will call the law office back in
a few days. Remember that you may need a signed release from patients
before you can say anything to people who approach you from outside
the clinical dyad.

Among the resources to help you with vexed issues of these sorts
are:

- Professional organizations, especially their listservs, where other
  therapists are typically happy to share their knowledge;

- Ethics committees or ethics experts in your discipline;

- The insurance agency providing your malpractice coverage (such
  companies employ attorneys who advise therapists at no charge);

- Consultation groups (peer supervision groups as well as those led
  by a senior consultant);

- Colleagues with experience in the relevant area;

- Current or former supervisors and consultants;

- Attorneys with expertise in mental health law.

You are not alone in such situations. You may practice solo all day and be used to making all the decisions for your practice, but these areas require more than clinical judgment. It is critical to remind yourself that you are not in fact an expert on issues that involve life beyond the consulting room. I find that therapists often feel they have an automatic responsibility to know everything applicable to their work and find a solution by themselves. Do not make that mistake. There is too much that we cannot know: laws change periodically, community standards differ from place to place, and no general training can apply to every professional challenge.

The second situation involves your own evaluation of your need for help. Your internal supervisor should get concerned, and urge you to get consultation from a trusted other, whenever you find that you recurrently feel a deep dread of meeting with a certain patient; when you find yourself ruminating about that person outside your business hours; when you repeatedly dream about a particular client; when you feel an overwhelming attraction to or disgust or hatred for a client; or when you repeatedly forget one person's appointments. Pay attention to any exceptions you find yourself making to how you ordinarily work. It is a red flag to notice that you are deviating from your usual professional norms in the case of one patient, however adequately you have rationalized that deviation (it may be clinically appropriate, but it is worth checking your thinking with someone you trust). At the highest level of internal red-flag-waving for seeking outside advice: When you cannot imagine telling another therapist what you said and did with a patient, it is time to do just that.

A trusted consultant might be the first source of help for what is going on between you and the client and what you might do to restore the therapeutic alliance and get the treatment moving. Intense countertransferences can be understood and alleviated by exposing them to people who know what it is like to feel chronically distorted or to be the object of a patient's relentless campaign of some sort. For this reason, therapists in Otto Kernberg's Personality Studies Institute meet weekly without fail (all participants, including Kernberg, present their hardest cases, a process he calls "intervision"). Simply because they are not in the midst of the emotional storms of your treatment, colleagues can offer perspectives that diminish your discomfort and suggest ways to handle the situation that have not occurred to you.

When both you and your client feel that your work together has become stalemated, you may be able to find a practitioner who will consult with you and the patient jointly to resolve the impasse. One outcome of the relational movement in psychoanalysis is that senior clinicians are increasingly comfortable with intervening with both parties in the therapy dyad (see Elkind, 1992). The comments of an external observer who knows how to avoid getting caught up in fault finding can reorient a treatment that has bogged down in mutual splitting and blaming. In some communities, this is still a new idea, so be careful to approach it tactfully.

If neither of these options is workable or effective, it may be time for you to see a therapist about what is going on in your own psyche or to talk about the issue with the therapist you already see. I discuss this problem-solving approach later in this chapter, with reference to instances when a current supervisor recommends that you talk with your therapist about an identified problem.

APPRECIATING THE SUPERVISOR'S SUBJECTIVITY

In all relationships, perhaps especially in those involving a power discrepancy, people easily misunderstand each other because they are interacting with internal objects more than the human being with whom they are engaged. In supervision, you will inevitably see your supervisor through a lens shaped by experiences and images of past authorities. This normal transference can be either mostly a blessing or mostly a curse. If you ordinarily felt secure with your early love objects, you will probably find yourself approaching supervision with some sense of safety, and in that emotional state you can explore your responses to being seen and evaluated. That is the blessing part. The curse part is that if prior caregivers and teachers were arbitrary, abusive, or negligent, posttraumatic reactions to authorities can interfere with your learning.

I should note that even if your early caregivers were paragons of support, your natural wish for their approval may have created a perfectionistic superego. This observation applies especially to oldest children (Sulloway, 1996), who are often attracted to the helping professions because they are used to taking care of younger siblings. Those of you who were firstborn have probably lamented that your parents were harder on you than on their subsequent children. You were the guinea pigs who slowly influenced them toward more reasonable expectations of their offspring. Oldest children have no big brother or sister to whom they can compare themselves; the fact that they hold themselves up to adult models creates in them lofty, often unrealistic, internal standards.

If you have been trying to live up to perfectionistic criteria, you may project your own excessive expectations onto anyone evaluating you and thus find yourself constantly anticipating negative supervisory judgment.

My experience has taught me that the best antidote to the effects of problematic childhood authorities and/or a harsh superego is a self-conscious attempt to differentiate your supervisor, at least intellectually, from the malignant influences in your past. In other words, you need to try to "mentalize" your supervisor (Fonagy & Target, 1996). Understanding where he or she is coming from, while questioning your automatic tendency to put any mentor in the generic category of "authority," may help you deal with problems that arise in your work together. Mentalization includes an appreciation of a person's traits and idiosyncrasies that may have little to do with who you are and how you behave. Depending on how self-disclosing your supervisor is, you may be able to learn a bit about the influences that gave rise to his or her style. Perhaps some qualities that you dislike are products of the supervisor's history and can even be understood in terms of his or her positive, adaptive efforts.

Mentalizing also involves an act of imagination about what it is like to inhabit a particular role. Roles themselves come with demands that can be usefully appreciated when you are in a reciprocal position. Irrespective of the power imbalance, the "goodness of fit" (Escalona, 1968; Rock, 1997) between you and your supervisor, your evaluation of your supervisor's skills as a mentor, or the realistic differences between the two of you in how you make sense of the clinical process, there are certain general features of supervisory responsibility that are likely part of your supervisor's motivation. There follow a few components of being a supervisor that may be germane.

Perhaps most important, individuals in supervisory roles tend to have a strong sense of responsibility. This internal inclination, a product of the overresponsible and self-critical dynamics I have mentioned in connection with the depressive temperaments of many clinicians, is strongly reinforced when a supervisor has actual legal responsibility for your patients. The burden of ultimate accountability for their welfare may make a mentor more critical or controlling than he or she would otherwise be. Try not to take it personally when your supervisor acts out of the anxiety that some action of yours may harm the clinical relationship or cause eventual problems that you may not have foreseen.

Second, in the supervisory role, clinicians have normal narcissistic needs to feel that they have given you something new, taken you a step further, and expanded your understanding. One of the reasons people like to supervise is that unlike psychodynamic work with patients, which requires constant care not to give personal opinions and advice, supervision offers the opportunity to say what one thinks and make recommendations about what the other person should do. When mentors pass their advice on to you, they can feel a sense of helpfulness that is more immediate and tangible that the longer-term rewards of patient care.

This need to feel effective in the supervisory hour can come into conflict with your own needs to feel seen, accepted, and validated. If you present your work hoping that your supervisor will simply bear witness to its excellence, and the supervisor instead suggests that you could have done something different, the experience can be deflating, especially if, in your prior educational experience, you were unambiguously a star. Good teachers and coaches typically nudge their mentees toward additional techniques, new angles of vision, and graduated levels of greater skill. You would be well advised to tell your fantasies of perfection to take a hike and to try to take in this novel paradigm of personal apprenticeship.

Third, part of a supervisor's job is to point out potential unintended consequences of interventions that your prior experience may have given you no reason to see as problematic. For example, you may be treating a woman with severe self-esteem deficits who asks you if you think of her as special. "Of course you are special!" you reply, leading from the heart, hoping your supervisor will consider this spontaneous reassurance an example of therapeutic empathy. Even if the mentor admires your loving attitude, it is a supervisory responsibility to bring up potential problems in well-intentioned statements. Your supervisor thus may suggest other possibilities for responding to your patient's question, such as asking why the question is coming up now, investigating ways the client's history made her feel profoundly *un*special, or hypothesizing that her need to be told she is special suggests that she has an internal problem with appreciating what is special in herself (otherwise, she would not need to ask), a problem that you and she can work to ameliorate.

The supervisor may point out that if reassurance from others were a reliable counteractive to low self-esteem, then friends and caring authorities in this woman's life would have already helped in that department, and she would not need psychotherapy. Instead of feeling an expansion of self-regard in the face of compliments, she may worry that people who deliver them are just trying to be kind. If this has been the case, the same assumption will arise in the treatment (e.g., via protestations that "You don't mean it; it's your job to be nice to me," or anxieties that she has duped you about her evident shortcomings, or idealizing worries that you are projecting your own specialness on to her rather than seeing her as she really is). Your mentor may go on to wonder if the patient will follow up with a test of her specialness, for example, by asking for a deviation from clinic policy that you are not authorized to give (e.g., being available by phone after clinic hours), by talking about her need for longer sessions, or by requesting that you read and discuss her poetry. It is not an attack to alert you to such possible outcomes and prepare you to deal with them. But it can feel like one if you incline toward self-criticism and thus tend to expect it from others.

Fourth, many psychoanalytic supervisors will see you as a potential colleague whom they look forward to welcoming into their community. They may expect to refer patients to you, and they may want to learn from you about any area in which you have more knowledge than they do. If your training program has been as infantilizing as many are, you may have lost sight of the fact that you are a competent adult, and this sudden shift to being treated as a fellow practitioner may be unsettling. I remember a supervisee who surprised me by being taken aback, and implying that I was trying to manipulate her, when I told someone who telephoned me during her supervisory hour, "I can't speak with you now; I'm consulting with a colleague." Keep this collegiality in mind when your supervisor asks you a question about your background and areas of interest or specialization. He or she may simply be trying to learn something from you. There may be no hidden agenda to expose something negative, as you may find yourself imagining.

Also remind yourself that even if the supervisor has extraordinary psychoanalytic intuition, he or she does not have x-ray vision. You need to talk about what you hope to get from working together. You should ask for clarification if you fail to understand something that the supervisor seems to assume you already get. If the atmosphere allows, you need to tell the supervisor when your feelings have been hurt. If the supervisor is not excessively narcissistic, he or she will want to know what helps and what does not. It can be aggravating for supervisors, who in fact admire a supervisee, to find themselves treated as potential persecutors rather than psychoanalytic compatriots.

In many clinical situations, your supervisor may suggest that you discuss a particular issue, often an intense countertransference reaction, with your own therapist. This is not a criticism of your overall mental health; it represents the supervisor's effort to keep from drifting into the role of treater rather than teacher. Psychoanalytic supervisors typically make such comments in the context of their own hard-won knowledge that patients often trigger aspects of our psyches that would not ordinarily be a focus of personal treatment. They make such recommendations in the spirit of assuming that we all take such issues to our personal therapists, not with an agenda to get you to see something particularly pathological about yourself.

MAXIMIZING THE VALUE OF LESS-THAN-IDEAL SUPERVISION

Supervisors are as diverse as clients, and the chemistry between the parties to a supervisory relationship is as critical as the fit between patient and therapist. You will probably have the bad luck to have at least one mentor who is not well suited to working with you, or who is inadequate or even destructive in some general way. Here are some ideas about how you may be able to deal with that situation.

First, try to find something of value in what the supervisor offers. Few human beings are utterly worthless. Letting a mentor know that you appreciate a positive feature of the supervision may go a long way, especially if he or she has not had the best experiences with supervisees in the past or has sensed that the chemistry between the two of you is less than ideal. Some years ago, because I had a patient with difficulties in the area of his research expertise, I took the risk of asking for a consultation with a prestigious academic colleague who had repeatedly made it clear that he thought most psychoanalytic therapists were idiots. To my surprise, despite his history of disdainful interruptions and other generally contemptuous treatment of me at faculty meetings, he warmed to our conversation when he saw that I had respect for his areas of superior knowledge. And I did in fact learn a lot from him (and interestingly, since then we have been on friendly terms). You may feel intimidated by a supervisor's power, but do not neglect the fact that there is a person behind it who needs ordinary validation and is trying to do good work.

If a supervisor gives you direction that you find confusing or unfamiliar (e.g., "Interpret resistance before content," "Use clarification followed by confrontation," "Don't interpret the idealization as a defense; just accept it," or "You have to get out of the doer–done-to position and open a third space"), ask for examples of putting the principle into practice. I remember an early supervisor who told me something like "analyze the transference as a split-off bad object from the paranoid–schizoid position." She clearly tended to think so automatically in the language of psychoanalytic object relations theory that she assumed I could easily do so as well. When I asked what she recommended that I should actually *say,* she clarified, "Tell him you think he's experiencing you as all bad, like the mother he often felt was entirely bad when he was very young." That was doable.

If you feel an ongoing tension between yourself and your supervisor, find a tactful way to bring it up. It may be readily addressable. If not, and you find that your supervisor reacts too defensively to make it possible to work the issue out between you, you have learned something about his or her limitations. You can later try framing the issue a different way and raising it in another context, but if this vessel also runs aground on the shoals of your supervisor's rigidity, it is time to accept that this person does not view supervision as a relationship that two people work together to improve. With any supervisor who believes that your job is to do exactly as directed, you have no choice but to put up with his or her mandates as best as you can.

Watch any tendency in yourself to act out, such as coming late to meetings, wearing dirty boots into the supervisor's office, forgetting to do paperwork you were asked to complete, or neglecting to read an article that your supervisor recommended. If your unconscious sabotages your best intentions, and you find that your behavior is expressing your negative feelings anyway, you should probably admit to your supervisor that you must have had some ambivalence of which you weren't conscious. There are many reasons for ambivalence in supervision, even when one is happy with a mentor, and few psychodynamic supervisors will treat such an admission as a major injury to their self-esteem. Confessing to an unconscious lapse is generally preferable to proffering excuses for actions that have erupted from your negative feelings.

In recent years, I have heard many examples of therapists in training who were being supervised by people who seemed to me to be less clinically skilled than the student. This may happen to you, and it may not be the last time you find yourself working for a boss with deficiencies in areas in which you are more talented or knowledgeable. The problem seems to occur most frequently in placements and internships in which experienced staff members are burned out by impossibly heavy caseloads and in which inexperienced staff are then put prematurely into supervisory positions because of the high personnel turnover created by such burnout. Try to talk back to the child in yourself who wants to protest that the grown-ups should be better than this, and make your peace with a disappointing reality.

If you have tried and failed to work things out with a supervisor, find out whether you can change to a different mentor. Obviously, if you are already in a position to choose your own supervisor, you can end the problematic relationship and sign up with someone else. If you are generally conflict avoidant, you may have to rehearse your comments ahead of time; for example, "Even though I admire many things about how you approach supervision, for some reason, this relationship doesn't seem to be going so well. I think it's time for me to see if someone else might be a better fit." If the supervisor is also feeling the incompatibility, he or she may be relieved.

If you are in a program that assigns supervisors to trainees, discuss your problem respectfully with the head of your training program and ask for a transfer. Perhaps other students have had similar complaints; if so, the faculty needs know that they may have to reconsider their appointment of this person to supervise their students. Many programs allow you to change supervisors if a relationship is not working out. If yours does not, you are in another situation in which you have to suck it up for a while and make the best of a bad deal.

On the topic of living with painful realities, it is not impossible to find yourself pathologized by organizational dynamics or by the blind spots of those in authority. You can get a reputation you do not deserve because a professor who misunderstands you primes how other faculty members regard you. I have occasionally known students who struck me as notably creative and prone to asking intellectually challenging questions who were treated this way. Such individuals are often inadequately prepared to deal with the expectations of some teachers that they be treated with more deference. Clinical environments may be different in this respect from some academic settings, where vigorous debate may be welcomed. If you are getting push-back from asking questions that are perceived as insubordinate, the most self-protective strategy would be to stop asking them.

Othering of this sort can also happen to students in minorities. Even programs that try to be sensitive to issues of diversity and privilege may have areas of ignorance that affect you. Research on students' experiences suggests that despite the self-representation of most teachers that they are enlightened about issues of diversity or lacking in prejudice and not given to stereotyping, in practice, many evidently do not sufficiently appreciate differences of class, culture, religion, sexuality, and other areas of identification (see Gomez, 2020). If you find yourself feeling misunderstood at a systems level, try to find a sympathetic person in authority to talk to about the problem. Fortunately, there is more support for you now, both in the professional literature and in professional associations, than there once was.

A supervisor external to your training program who reports positively to the faculty on your clinical work can help to prune prejudices against you that may have taken root there, but sometimes the reputation you had in your program will linger. I was consulted not long ago by a man whose initial supervisor wrongly perceived him as flirting with female patients and shared his misgivings with faculty members in the student's program. This young therapist was gay (he thought obviously so); he had been trying to inject a playful note into working with two women whom he saw as emotionally deadened. But under the influence of their colleague, the faculty construed him as tending to "act out" with clients, and this characterization had followed him to his internship. I advised him to talk directly to his supervisor there about his own version of the story. Although systemic othering is hard to counteract, it is not a life sentence. You may need to remind yourself that you are not completely helpless when you find yourself the object of microaggressions you do not deserve, and that your professional community will eventually judge you on your own merits.

WHEN THE PROBLEM IS YOU

In what I have written so far, I am assuming that most readers are sensitive, well intentioned, inclined toward self-criticism, and easily wounded by negative attributions. My graduate students, who have almost all struck me as excellent natural therapists, tend to be quick to think that anything that goes wrong between them and their patients, or between them and their mentors, is their own "fault." It is my impression that most of them tend to believe they are guilty whenever they are criticized and are consequently slow to realize that a recurrent problem may reflect on a supervisor or program rather than on themselves. So my advice so far has tilted in the direction of helping you keep a legitimately positive opinion of yourself.

Most of us, however, also have some personal dynamics that can reduce the effectiveness of our clinical work. Some of us have one or two areas that we need to deal with before we can work well with certain clinical challenges. Although I have occasionally encountered psychodynamic clinicians who seem to be gifted and mentally healthy enough to be fine therapists without personal treatment, most of us need it, and in the right therapeutic dyad, all of us can profit from it. (I note here that there are a few aspiring clinicians who simply should not be therapists;

for them, no amount of their own psychotherapy will turn them into skilled practitioners. These people do need to rethink their careers.)

If you keep getting negative feedback about your clinical capacities, especially from more than one supervisor, and you cannot seem to find a way to change the perception of those who work with you, it is time to take a hard look at yourself. If you are not already in therapy, go into treatment with someone you know to be thoughtful and experienced, with whom you feel comfortable talking openly. Do this even if it stresses you out financially. There is nothing more important than confronting problems in your own psychology that keep coming up in your clinical work.

Even if other issues predominate in your personal treatment, make space there to talk about any negative feedback you are getting from supervisors. If they are accurately attuned to your own conflicts, your therapist should be able to explore the problematic issues with you, because the same interpersonal dynamics will almost certainly come into your therapeutic relationship. Dealing with them in treatment can prevent their causing trouble elsewhere. With help from your therapist, you may be able to change the personal qualities that trouble your supervisors. If such change seems unattainable, you may have to use your therapy to consider what kinds of patients or situations you should avoid in the future, on the basis that they tend to activate your own vulnerabilities.

CONCLUDING COMMENTS

I hope this chapter's ideas and advice will help you maximize the value of whatever supervision and consultation you are receiving or will soon receive. I have attested to the importance of supervisory relationships both for handling immediate clinical challenges and for preparing you for a long career as a psychotherapist. I have emphasized the process of developing your own internal supervisory voice as well as your sense of when you should go for consultation, irrespective of how many years ago you were credentialed. I have encouraged you to empathize with your mentor's perspective and, in doing so, tried to provide a counterweight to the tendency we all have to project our earlier experiences of authority into the supervision scenario.

Finally, I have discussed some circumstances in which your supervisory experience may fall short of your expectations and hopes, whether because of limitations in your supervisor, a poor fit between you and the supervisor, systemic dynamics, external pressures antithetical to your training needs, or your own psychological challenges. Fortunately, as you become more and more experienced, you will have increasing freedom to manage your own ongoing learning, and you will know better what you need from mentors and consultants. Even a bad early start can be counteracted by later experience with positive supervisory relationships.

References

Abbass, A. (2004). A small-group videotape training for psychotherapy skills development. *Academic Psychiatry, 28,* 151–155.

Abbass, A. (2016). The emergence of psychodynamic psychotherapy for treatment resistant patients: Intensive short-term dynamic psychotherapy. *Psychodynamic Psychiatry, 44*(2), 245–280.

Abbass, A., Kisely, S. R., Town, J. M., Leichsenring, F., Driessen, E., De Maat, S., . . . Crowe, E. (2014). Short-term psychodynamic psychotherapies for common mental disorders. *Cochrane Database of Systematic Reviews,* Issue 4, Article No. CD004687.

Abbass, A. A., Rabung, S., Leichsenring, F., Refseth, J., & Midgley, N. (2013). Psychodynamic psychotherapy for children and adolescents: A meta-analysis of short-term psychodynamic models. *Journal of the American Academy of Child and Adolescent Psychiatry, 52*(8), 863–875.

Abrevaya, E., & Thomson-Salo, F. (Eds.). (2019). *Homosexualities: Psychogenesis, polymorphism, and countertransference.* New York: Routledge.

Ackerman, S. J., & Hilsenroth, M. J. (2003). A review of therapist characteristics and techniques positively impacting the therapeutic alliance. *Clinical Psychology Review, 23*(1), 1–33.

Aggarwal, P., & Bhatia, P. (2020). Clinical supervision in forensic psychiatry in India. *Journal of Psychotherapy Integration, 30*(1), 9–15.

Ainslie, R. (2011). Immigration and the psychodynamics of class. *Psychoanalytic Psychology, 28*(4), 560–568.

Ainsworth, M. D. S., & Bell, S. M. (1970). Attachment, exploration, and separation: Illustrated by the behavior of one-year-olds in a strange situation. *Child Development, 41*(1), 49–67.

Akhtar, S. (Ed.). (2014). *The African American experience: Psychoanalytic perspectives.* New York: Rowman & Littlefield.

Allison, E., & Fonagy, P. (2016). When is truth relevant? *Psychoanalytic Quarterly, 85*(2), 275–303.

Alonso, A. (1985). *The quiet profession: Supervision of psychotherapy.* New York: Macmillan.

American Psychological Association. (2012). Recognition of psychotherapy effectiveness. Retrieved from *www.apa.org/about/policy/resolution-psychotherapy.aspx.*

American Psychological Association. (2017). Ethical principles of psychologists and code of conduct (2002, amended effective June 1, 2010, and January 1, 2017). Retrieved from *www.apa.org/ethics /code/index.aspx.*

Anstadt, T., Merten, J., Ullrich, B., & Krause, R. (1997). Affective dyadic behavior, core conflictual relationship themes and success of treatment. *Psychotherapy Research, 7*(4), 397–417.

Arkowitz, S. W. (2001). Perfectionism in the supervisee. In S. Gill (Ed.), *The supervisory alliance: Facilitating the psychotherapist's learning experience* (pp. 3–66). Northvale, NJ: Jason Aronson.

Arlow, J. (1972). Some dilemmas in psychoanalytic education. *Journal of the American Psychoanalytic Association, 20*(3), 556–566.

Aron, L. (1991). The patient's experience of the analyst's subjectivity. *Psychoanalytic Dialogues, 1*(1), 29–51.

Aronson, S. (2000). Analytic supervision: All work and no play? *Contemporary Psychoanalysis, 36*(1), 121–132.

Auchincloss, E. L., & Michels, R. (2003). A reassessment of psychoanalytic education: Controversies and changes. *International Journal of Psychoanalysis, 84*(2), 387–403.

Auchincloss, E. L., & Weiss, R. W. (1992). Paranoid character and the intolerance of indifference. *Journal of the American Psychoanalytic Association, 40*(4), 1013–1037.

Auerbach, J. S. (2019). Relatedness, self-definition, mental representation, and internalization in the work of Sidney J. Blatt: Scientific and clinical contributions. *Psychoanalytic Psychology, 35*(4), 291–302.

Balint, M. (1948). On the psycho-analytic training system. *International Journal of Psychoanalysis, 29,* 163–173.

Baltes, P. B., Glück, J., & Kunzmann, U. (2002). Wisdom: Its structure and function in regulating successful lifespan development. In C. R. Snyder & S. J. Lopez (Eds.), *Handbook of positive psychology* (pp. 327–347). New York: Oxford University Press.

Bambling, M. (2000). The effect of clinical supervision on the development of counsellor competency. *Psychotherapy in Australia, 6*(4), 58–63.

Barlow, J., Bennett, C., Midgley, N., Larkin, S., & Wei, Y. (2015). Parent–infant psychotherapy for improving parental and infant mental health. *Cochrane Database of Systematic Reviews,* Issue 1, Article No. CD010534.

Bateman, A., & Fonagy, P. (2013). Mentalization-based treatment. *Psychoanalytic Inquiry, 33*(6), 595–613.

Battan, J. (1983). The "new narcissism" in 20th-century America: The shadow and substance of social change. *Journal of Social History, 17*(2), 199–220.

Baudry, F. D. (1993). The personal dimension and management of the supervisory situation with a special note on the parallel process. *Psychoanalytic Quarterly, 62*(4), 588–614.

Baum-Baicker, C. (2018). Defining clinical wisdom part II: Quotes, the qualitative underpinning of the research. *JASPER International: Journal for the Advancement of Scientific Psychoanalytic Empirical Research, 2*(1), 105–118.

Baum-Baicker, C., & Sisti, D. W. *(*2012). Clinical wisdom in psychoanalysis and psychodynamic psychotherapy: A philosophical and qualitative analysis. *Journal of Clinical Ethics, 23*(1), 13–40.

Beebe, B., & Lachmann, F. (2014). *The origins of attachment: Infant research and adult attachment.* New York: Routledge.

Beitman, B. D., & Yue, D. (2004). *Learning psychotherapy* (2nd ed.). New York: Norton.

Bellak, L., Hurvich, M., & Gediman, H. K. (1973). *Ego functions in schizophrenics, neurotics, and normals: A systematic study of conceptual, diagnostic, and therapeutic aspects.* New York: Wiley.

Benedek, T., & Fleming, J. (1983). *Psychoanalytic supervision: A model of clinical training.* New York: International Universities Press.

Benjamin, J. (2017). *Beyond doer and done to: Recognition theory, intersubjectivity and the third.* New York: Routledge.

Berman, E. (2000). Psychoanalytic supervision: The intersubjective development. *International Journal of Psychoanalysis, 81*(2), 273–290.

Berman, E. (2001). Psychoanalytic supervision at the crossroads. In S. Gill (Ed.), *The supervisory alliance: Facilitating the psychotherapist's learning experience* (pp. 161–186). Northvale, NJ: Jason Aronson.

Berman, J., & Mosher, P. W. (2019). Part One: Sexual boundary violations. In *Off the tracks: Cautionary tales about the derailing of mental health care* (Vol. 1, pp. 1–314). New York: International Psychoanalytic Books.

Bernard, J. M., & Goodyear, R. K. (2009). *Fundamentals of clinical supervision* (4th ed.). Upper Saddle River, NJ: Merrill.

Bernard, J. M., & Goodyear, R. K. (2018). *Fundamentals of clinical supervision* (6th ed.). New York: Pearson.

Bernfeld, S. (1962). On psychoanalytic training. *Psychoanalytic Quarterly, 31*(4), 453–421.

Bernhardt, I. S., Nissen-Lie, H., Moltu, C., McLeod, J., & Råbu, M. (2019). "It's both a strength and a drawback." How therapists' personal qualities are experienced in their professional work. *Psychotherapy Research, 29*(7), 959–970.

Bion, W. R. (1961). *Experiences in groups.* New York: Basic Books.

Bion, W. R. (1962). *Learning from experience.* London: Heinemann.

Birkhofer, C. (2017). Theoretical diversity and pluralism in psychoanalysis: Change, challenges, and benefits. *Psychoanalytic Psychology, 34*(1), 114–121.

Blagys, M. D., & Hilsenroth, M. J. (2000). Distinctive of short-term psychodynamic-interpersonal psychotherapy: A review of the comparative psychotherapy process literature. *Clinical Psychology: Science and Practice, 7*(2), 167–189.

Blatt, S. J. (2008). *Polarities of experience: Relatedness and self-definition in personality development, psychopathology, and the therapeutic process.* Washington, DC: American Psychological Association.

Bollas, C. (1987). *The shadow of the object.* London: Free Association Books.

Bollas, C., & Sundelson, D. (1995). *The new informants: The betrayal of confidentiality in psychoanalysis and psychotherapy.* Northvale, NJ: Jason Aronson.

Bonovitz, C. (2010). What is "good technique? How to teach it? Personal reflections on psychoanalytic training. *American Journal of Psychoanalysis, 70*(1), 65–77.

Bowlby, J. (1969). *Attachment and loss: Vol. I. Attachment.* New York: Basic Books.

Bowlby, J. (1973). *Attachment and loss: Vol. II. Separation: anxiety and anger.* New York: Basic Books.

Boyd-Franklin, N., Cleek, E. N., Wofsky, M., & Mundy, B. (2015). *Therapy in the real world: Effective treatments for challenging problems.* New York: Guilford Press.

Brenner, A., & Khan, F. (2013). The training of psychodynamic psychiatrists: The concept of "psychoanalytic virtue." *Psychodynamic Psychiatry, 41*(1), 57–74.

Bromberg, P. M. (1998). *Standing in the spaces: Essays on clinical process, trauma and dissociation.* Hillsdale, NJ: Analytic Press.

Brothers, D. (2014). Traumatic attachments: Intergenerational trauma, dissociation, and the analytic relationship. *International Journal of Psychoanalytic Self Psychology, 9*(1), 3–15.

Brown, C. (2010). Perspectives on difference in psychoanalytic supervision. *Attachment: New Directions in Psychotherapy and Relational Psychoanalysis, 4*(3), 275–287.

Bruzzone, M., Casaula, E., Jimenez, J. P., & Jordan, J. F. (1985). Regression and persecution in analytic training. Reflections on experience. *International Review of Psychoanalysis, 12,* 411–415.

Buber, M. (1937). *I and thou.* New York: Charles Scribner's Sons.

Bucci, W., & Maski, B. (2007). Beneath the surface of the therapeutic interaction: The psychoanalytic method in modern dress. *Journal of the American Psychoanalytic Association, 55*(4), 1355–1397.

Buchheim, A., Viviani, R., Kessler, H., Kachele, H., Cierpka, M., Roth, G., . . . Taubner, S. (2012, March 28). Changes in prefrontal-limbic function in major depression after 15 months of long-term psychotherapy. *Plos ONE, 7*(3), e33745.

Buechler, S. (2004). *Clinical values: Emotions that guide psychoanalytic treatment.* Hillsdale, NJ: Analytic Press.

Cabaniss, D. L., Glick, R. A., & Roose, S. P. (2001). The Columbia Supervision Project: Data from the dyad. *Journal of the American Psychoanalytic Association 49*(1), 235–267.

Cabaniss, D. L., & Roose, S. P. (1997). The control case: A unique analytic situation. *Journal of the American Psychoanalytic Association, 45*(1), 189–199.

Cabaniss, D. L., Schein, J. W., Rosen, P., & Roose, S. P. (2003). Candidate progress in psychoanalytic institutes: A multicentric study. *International Journal of Psychoanalysis, 84*(1), 77–94.

Cain, S. (2012). *Quiet: The power of introverts in a world that can't stop talking.* New York: Crown.

Calef, V., & Weinshel, E. (1981). Some clinical consequences of introjection: Gaslighting. *Psychoanalytic Quarterly, 50*(1), 44–66.

Caligor, E., Kernberg, O. F., Clarkin, J. F., & Yeomans, F. E. (2018). *Psychodynamic therapy for personality pathology: Treating self and interpersonal functioning.* Washington, DC: American Psychiatric Association.

Caligor, L. (1981). Parallel and reciprocal processes in psychoanalytic supervision. *Contemporary Psychoanalysis, 17*(1), 1–27.

Caligor, L., Bromberg, P., & Meltzer, J. (1984). *Clinical perspectives in the supervision of psychoanalysis and psychotherapy.* New York: Plenum Press.

Callahan, J. L. (Ed.). (2020). Supervisee perspectives of supervision process [Special Issue]. *Journal of Psychotherapy Integration, 30*(1).

Callahan, J. L., & Love, P. K. (2019). Supervisee perspectives on supervision processes [Special Issue]. *Training and Education in Professional Psychology, 13*(3).

Campos, R. C. (2013). Conceptualization and preliminary validation of a depressive personality concept. *Psychoanalytic Psychology, 30*(4), 601–620.

Casement, P. J. (1985). *Learning from the patient.* New York: Guilford Press.

Casement, P. J. (2002). *Learning from our mistakes: Beyond dogma in psychoanalysis and psychotherapy.* New York: Guilford Press.

Casement, P. J. (2005). The emperor's clothes: Some serious problems in psychoanalytic training. *International Journal of Psychoanalysis, 86*(4), 1143–1160.

Cassidy, J., & Shaver, P. R. (Eds.). (2016). *Handbook of attachment: Theory, research, and clinical applications.* New York: Guilford Press.

Castonguay, L. G., & Hill, C. E. (Eds.). (2007). *Insight in psychotherapy.* Washington, DC: American Psychological Association.

Celenza, A. (2011). *Sexual boundary violations: Therapeutic, supervisory, and academic contexts.* Northvale, NJ: Jason Aronson.

Chefetz, R. A. (2015). *Intensive psychotherapy for persistent dissociative processes: The fear of feeling real.* New York: Norton.

Coburn, W. J. (2001). Transference–countertransference dynamics and disclosure in supervision. In S. Gill (Ed.), *The supervisory alliance: Facilitating the psychotherapist's learning experience* (pp. 215–232). Northvale, NJ: Jason Aronson.

Corbett, K. (2011). *Boyhoods: Rethinking masculinities.* New Haven, CT: Yale University Press.

Craig, A. D. (2009). How do you feel – now? The anterior insula and human awareness. *Nature Reviews: Neuroscience, 10*(1), 59–70.

Cucco, E. (2020). Who's afraid of the big bad unconscious: Working with countertransference in training. *Journal of Psychotherapy Integration, 30*(1), 52–59.

Davids, M. F. (2011). *Internal racism: A psychoanalytic approach.* London: Red Globe Press.

Davis, L. J. (1995). *Enforcing normalcy: Disability, deafness and the body.* New York: Verso.

De Masi, F. (2019). Essential elements of the work of a supervisor. *American Journal of Psychoanalysis 79*(3), 388–397.

De Smet, M. M., Reitske, M., De Geest, R., Norman, U. A., Truijens, F., & Desmet, M. (2020). What "good outcome" means to patients: Understanding recovery and improvement in psychotherapy for major depression from a mixed-methods perspective. *Journal of Counseling Psychology, 67*(1), 25–29.

Deutsch, H. (1942). Some forms of emotional disturbance and their relationship to schizophrenia. *Psychoanalytic Quarterly, 11*(3), 301–321.

Dewald, P. A. (1987). *Learning process in psychoanalytic supervision: Challenges and complexities.* Madison, CT: International Universities Press.

Diener, M. J., & Mesrie, V. (2015). Supervisory process from a supportive-expressive relational psychodynamic approach. *Psychotherapy, 52*(2), 153–157.

Dimen, M. (2014). *Sexuality, intimacy, power.* New York: Routledge.

Doehrman, M. (1976). Parallel processes in supervision and psychotherapy. *Bulletin of the Menninger Clinic, 40*(1), 3–104.

Drescher, J. (2002). Don't ask, don't tell: A gay man's perspective on the psycho-analytic training between 1973 and 1991. *Journal of Gay & Lesbian Psycho-therapy, 6*(1), 45–55.

Drescher, J. (2015). Out of DSM: Depathologizing homosexuality. *Behavioral Science, 5*, 565–575.

Drescher, J., & Fors, M. (2018). An appreciation and critique of PDM-2's focus on minority stress through the case of Frank. *Psychoanalytic Psychology, 35*(3), 357–362.

Driessen, E., Hegelmaier, L. M., Abbass, A. A., Barber, J. P., Dekker, J. J. M., Van, H. L., . . . Cuijpers, P. (2015). The efficacy of short-term psychodynamic psychotherapy for depression: A meta-analysis update. *Clinical Psychology Review, 42*(Dec.), 1–15.

Dulchin, J., & Segal, A. (1982a). The ambiguity of confidentiality in a psychoanalytic institute. *Psychiatry, 45*(1), 13–25.

Dulchin, J., & Segal, A. (1982b). Third party confidences: The uses of information in a psychoanalytic institute. *Psychiatry, 45*(1), 27–37.

Eagle, G., & Long, C. (2014). Supervision of psychoanalytic/psychodynamic psychotherapy. In C. E. Watkins, Jr., & D. L. Milne (Eds.), *The Wiley international handbook of clinical supervision* (pp. 471–492). Malden, MA: Wiley Blackwell.

Eagle, M. N. (2013). *Attachment and psychoanalysis: Theory, research, and implications.* New York: Guilford Press.

Edwards, J. (2011). *The sibling relationship: A force for growth and conflict.* New York: Jason Aronson.

Ehrensaft, D. (2014). Listening and learning from gender-nonconforming children. *Psychoanalytic Study of the Child, 68*, 28–56.

Eigen, M. (1981). The area of faith in Winnicott, Lacan and Bion. *International Journal of Psychoanalysis, 62*, 413–433.

Eisold, K. (2000). Review of *Unfree associations: Inside psychoanalytic institutes* by Douglas Kirsner. *Free Associations, 8*(2), 170–172.

Eisold, K. (2004). Psychoanalytic training: The "faculty system." *Psychoanalytic Inquiry, 24*(1), 51–70.

Eitingon, M. (1923). Report of the Berlin Psychoanalytical Policlinic. *International Journal of Psychoanalysis, 4*, 254–269.

Eitingon, M. (1926). Report on the Ninth International Psychoanalytic Congress. *International Journal of Psychoanalysis, 7*, 130–134.

Ekstein, R., & Wallerstein, R. S. (1958; rev. ed. 1971). *The teaching and learning of psychotherapy.* Madison, CT: International Universities Press.

Elkind, S. N. (1992). *Resolving impasses in therapeutic relationships.* New York: Guilford Press.

Ellis, M. V. (2017). Narratives of harmful clinical supervision. *The Clinical Supervisor, 36*(1), 20–87.

Ellis, M. V., Berman, L., Hanus, A. E., Swords, B. A., Ayala, E. E., & Siembor, M. (2014). Inadequate and harmful clinical supervision: Testing a revised framework and assessing occurrence. *The Counseling Psychologist, 42*(4), 434–472.

Ericssson, K. A., Krampe, R. T., & Tesch-Römer, C. (1993). The role of deliberate practice in the acquisition of expert performance. *Psychological Review, 100*(3), 363–406.

Erikson, E. (1950). *Childhood and society.* New York: Norton.

Erikson, E. (1968). *Identity: Youth and crisis.* New York: Norton.

Erle, J. B. (1979). An approach to the study of analyzability and analyses: The course of forty consecutive cases selected for supervised analysis. *Psychoanalytic Quarterly, 48*(2), 198–228.

Escalona, S. K. (1968). *The roots of individuality: Normal patterns of development in infancy.* Chicago: Aldine.

Eubanks, C. F., Muran, J. C., Dreher, D., Sergi, M. A., Silberstein, E., & Wasserman, M. (2019). Trainees' experiences in alliance-focused training: The risks and rewards of learning to negotiate ruptures. *Psychoanalytic Psychology, 36*(2), 122–131.

Evans, M. (2011). Pinned against the ropes: Understanding anti-social personality-disordered patients through use of the counter-transference. *Psychoanalytic Psychotherapy, 25*(2), 143-156.

Falender, C. A., & Shafranske, E. P. (2016). *Supervision essentials for the practice of competency-based supervision.* Washington, DC: American Psychoanalytic Association.

Feinstein, R. E. (2020). Descriptions and reflections on the cognitive apprenticeship model of psychotherapy training and supervision. *Journal of Contemporary Psychotherapy.* [Epub ahead of print]

Feinstein, R. E., Huhn, R., & Yaeger, J. (2015). Apprenticeship model of psychotherapy training and supervision: Utilizing six tools of experiential learning. *Academic Psychiatry, 39*(5), 585–589.

Feinstein, R. E., & Yager, J. (2013). Advanced psychotherapy training: Psychotherapy scholars' track, and the apprenticeship model. *Academic Psychiatry, 37*(1), 248–253.

Firestein, S. (1978). *Termination in psychoanalysis.* New York: International Universities Press.

Fleming, J., & Benedek, T. (1966). *Psychoanalytic supervision.* New York: Grune & Stratton.

Flückiger, C., Del Re, A. C., Wampold, B. E., Symonds, D., & Horvath, A. O. (2012). How central is the alliance in psychotherapy?: A multilevel longitudinal meta-analysis. *Journal of Counseling Psychology, 59*(1), 10–17.

Fonagy, P., & Allison, E. (2016). Commentary on Kernberg and Michels. *Journal of the American Psychoanalytic Association, 64*(3), 495–500.

Fonagy, P., & Target, M. (1996). Playing with reality: I. Theory of mind and the development of psychic reality. *International Journal of Psychoanalysis, 77,* 217–223.

Fors, M. (2018). *A grammar of power in psychotherapy: Exploring the dynamics of privilege.* Washington, DC: American Psychological Association.

Fors, M., & McWilliams, N. (2016). Collaborative reading of medical records in psychotherapy: A feminist psychoanalytic proposal about narrative and empowerment. *Psychoanalytic Psychology, 33*(1), 35–57.

Fosha, D. (2005). Emotion, true self, true other, core state: Toward a clinical theory of affective change process. *Psychoanalytic Review, 92*(4), 513–551.

Foster, R. P., Moskowitz, M., & Javier, R. A. (Eds.). (1996). *Reaching across boundaries of culture and class: Widening the scope of psychotherapy.* Northvale, NJ: Jason Aronson.

Frank, K. (2001). Expanding the field of psychoanalytic change: Exploratory-asser-
tive motivation, self-efficacy, and the new analytic role for action. *Psychoanalytic Inquiry, 21(5)*, 620–639.

Frawley-O'Dea, M. G., & Sarnat, J. E. (2000). *The supervisory relationship: A contemporary psychodynamic approach*. New York: Guilford Press.

Freud, A. (1938). The problem of training analysis. In *The writings of Anna Freud*
(pp. 407–421). New York: International Universities Press, 1968.

Freud, S. (1896). Further remarks on the neuro-psychoses of defence. *Standard Edition, 3*, 162–185.

Freud, S. (1911a). The handling of dream-interpretation in psycho-analysis. *Standard Edition, 12*, 89–96.

Freud, S. (1911b). Psychoanalytic notes on an autobiographical account of a case of
paranoia. *Standard Edition, 12*, 3–82.

Freud, S. (1912a). The dynamics of transference. *Standard Edition, 12*, 97–108.

Freud, S. (1912b). Recommendations to physicians practicing psycho-analysis. *Standard Edition, 12*, 109–120.

Freud, S. (1913). On beginning the treatment (Further recommendations on the
technique of psycho-analysis I). *Standard Edition, 12*, 121–142.

Freud, S. (1914). Remembering, repeating and working-through (Further recommendations on the technique of psycho-analysis II). *Standard Edition, 12*,
143–156.

Freud, S. (1915). Observations on transference-love (Further recommendations on
the technique of psycho-analysis III). *Standard Edition, 12*, 157–171.

Freud, S. (1920). Beyond the pleasure principle. *Standard Edition, 18*, 7–64.

Freud, S. (1923). The ego and the id. *Standard Edition, 12*, 1–66.

Freud, S. (1926). The question of lay analysis: Conversations with an impartial person. *Standard Edition, 20*, 183–258.

Freud, S. (1937). Analysis terminable and interminable. *Standard Edition, 28*, 209–
254.

Frijling-Schreuder, E. (1970). On individual supervision. *International Journal of
Psychoanalysis, 51(2)*, 363–370.

Frosch, A. (2006). The culture of psychoanalysis and the concept of analyzability.
Psychoanalytic Psychology, 23(1), 43–55.

Furlong, A. (2005). Confidentiality with respect to third parties: A psychoanalytic
view. *International Journal of Psychoanalysis, 86(2)*, 375–394.

Gabbard, G. O. (1995). The early history of boundary violations in psychoanalysis.
Journal of the American Psychoanalytic Association, 43(4), 1115–1136.

Gabbard, G. O. (2016). *Boundaries and boundary violations in psychoanalysis*.
Washington, DC: American Psychiatric Association.

Gard, D. E., & Lewis, J. M. (2008). Building the supervisory alliance with beginning therapists. *The Clinical Supervisor, 27(1)*, 39–60.

Garfield, D., & Havens, L. (1991). Paranoid phenomena and pathological narcissism. *American Journal of Psychotherapy, 45(2)*, 160–172.

Garrett, M. (2019). *Psychotherapy for psychosis: Integrating cognitive-behavioral
and psychodynamic treatment*. New York: Guilford Press.

Gartner, R. B. (2014). Trauma and countertrauma, resilience and counterresilience.
Contemporary Psychoanalysis, 50(4), 609–626.

Gediman, H. K., & Wolkenfeld, F. (1980). The parallelism phenomenon in psychoanalytic supervision: Its reconsideration as a triadic system. *Psychoanalytic Quarterly, 49*(2), 234–255.

Geller, J. D., Farber, B. A., & Schaffer, C. E. (2010). Representations of the supervisory dialogue and the development of psychotherapists. *Psychotherapy: Theory, Research, Practice, Training, 47*(2), 211–220.

Geller, J. D., Norcross, J. C., & Orlinsky, D. E. (Eds.). (2005). *The psychotherapist's own psychotherapy: Patient and clinician perspectives*. New York: Oxford University Press.

Gentile, J. (2018). *Freud, free speech, and the voice of desire*. New York: Routledge.

Ghent, E. (1990). Masochism, submission, surrender—Masochism as a perversion of surrender. *Contemporary Psychoanalysis, 26*(1), 108–136.

Gherovici, P., & Christian, C. (2018). *Psychoanalysis in the barrios: Race, class, and the unconscious*. New York: Routledge.

Gill, S. (1999). Narcissistic vulnerability in psychoanalytic supervisees: Ego ideals, self-exposure and narcissistic character defenses. *International Forum of Psychoanalysis, 8*(3–4), 227–232.

Gill, S. (Ed.) (2001), *The supervisory alliance: Facilitating the psychotherapist's learning experience*. Northvale, NJ: Jason Aronson.

Gilligan, C. (1982). *In a different voice: Psychological theory and women's development*. Cambridge, MA: Harvard University Press.

Gilligan, J. (1996). *Violence: Our deadly epidemic and its causes*. New York: Putnam.

Ginsberg, K. R. (2014). *Building resilience in children and teens: Giving kids roots and wings* (2nd ed.). Elk Grove Village, IL: American Academy of Pediatrics.

Gladwell, M. (2011). *Outliers: The story of success*. New York: Little, Brown.

Gomez, J. M. (2020). Training perspectives on relational cultural therapy and cultural competency in supervision of trauma cases. *Journal of Psychotherapy Integration, 30*(1), 60–66.

Grand, S., & Salberg, J. (Eds.). (2017). *Trans-generational trauma and the other: Dialogues across history and difference*. New York: Routledge.

Gray, L. A., Ladany, N., Walker, J. A., & Ancis, J. R. (2001). Psychotherapy trainees' experience of counterproductive events in supervision. *Journal of Counseling Psychology, 48*(4), 371–383.

Greedharry, M. (2008). *Postcolonial theory and psychoanalysis*. New York: Palgrave Macmillan.

Green, A. (1993). *Le travail du négative*. Paris: Editions de Minuit.

Greenacre, P. (1954). The role of transference—Practical considerations in relation to psychoanalytic therapy. *Journal of the American Psychoanalytic Association, 2*(4), 671–684.

Greenberg, L. S. (2014). The therapeutic relationship in emotion-focused therapy. *Psychotherapy, 51*(3), 350–357.

Gregory, R. J., & Remen, A. L. (2008). A manual-based psychodynamic therapy for treatment-resistant borderline personality disorder. *Psychotherapy: Theory, Research, Practice, Training, 45*(1), 15–27.

Gregus, S. J., Stevens, K. T., Sievert, N. P., Tucker, R. P., & Callahan, J. L. (2020). Student perceptions of multicultural training and program climate in clinical psychology and doctoral programs. *Training and Education in Professional Psychology, 14*(4), 293–307.

Guest, P. D., & Beutler, L. E. (1988). Impact of psychotherapy supervision on therapist orientation and values. *Journal of Counseling and Clinical Psychology*, *56*(5), 653–658.

Guntrip, H. (1969). *Schizoid phenomena, object relations and the self*. New York: International Universities Press.

Hanoch, E. (2006). The loudness of the unspoken: Candidates' anxiety in supervision. *Psychoanalytic Perspectives*, *3*(2), 127–146.

Harrell, S. P. (2014). Compassionate confrontation and empathic exploration: The integration of race-related narratives in clinical supervision. In C. Falender (Ed.), *Multiculturalism and diversity in clinical supervision: A competency-based approach* (pp. 82–112). Washington, DC: American Psychological Association.

Harris, A. (2008). *Gender as soft assembly*. New York: Routledge.

Hart, A., Dunn, J., & Jones, L. (2020). A preview of how psychoanalytic training institutes are addressing the diversities. *The American Psychoanalyst*, *54*(3), 14, 18–19.

Hawkins, P., & Shohet, R. (2012). *Supervision in the helping professions* (4th ed.). Maidenhead, Berkshire, UK: Open University Press.

Hayes, J. A., Gelso, C. J., Goldberg, S., & Kivlighan, D. M. (2018). Countertransference management and effective psychotherapy: Meta-analytic findings. *Psychotherapy*, *55*(4), 496–507.

Helbig-Lang, S., & Petermann, F. (2010). Tolerate or eliminate? A systematic review on the effects of safety behavior across anxiety disorders. *Clinical Psychology: Science and Practice*, *17*(3), 218–233.

Henry, W. P., Schacht, T. E., Strupp, H. H., Butler, S. F., & Binder, J. L. (1993). Effects of training in time-limited dynamic psychotherapy: Mediators of therapists' responses to training. *Journal of Consulting and Clinical Psychology*, *61*(3), 441–447.

Hess, A. K., Hess, K. D., & Hess, T. H. (2008). *Psychotherapy supervision: Theory, research and practice*. New York: Wiley.

Høglend, P., Amlo, S., Marble, A., Bøgwald, K-P., Sørbye, Ø., Sjaastad, M. C., & Heyderdahl, O. (2006). Analysis of the patient-therapist relationship in dynamic psychotherapy: An experimental study of transference interpretations. *American Journal of Psychiatry*, *164*(10), 1739–1746.

Holmes, D. E. (1992). Race and transference in psychoanalysis and psychotherapy. *International Journal of Psychoanalysis*, *73*(1), 1–11.

Holmes, D. E. (2016). Culturally imposed trauma: The sleeping dog has awakened. Will psychoanalysis take heed? *Psychoanalytic Dialogues*, *26*(6), 641–654.

Horney, H. (1950). *Neurosis and human growth: The struggle toward self-realization*. New York: Norton.

Howell, E. (2020). *Trauma and dissociation informed psychotherapy: Relational healing and the therapeutic connection*. New York: Norton.

Huprich, S. (1998). Depressive personality disorder: Theoretical issues, clinical findings, and future research questions. *Clinical Psychology Review*, *18*(5), 477–500.

Huprich, S. (2014). Malignant self-regard: A self-structure enhancing the understanding of masochistic, depressive, and vulnerably narcissistic personalities. *Harvard Review of Psychiatry*, *22*(5), 293–305.

Hyde, J. (2009). *Fragile narcissists or the guilty good. What drives the personality of the psychotherapist?* Unpublished doctoral dissertation, Macquarie University, Sydney, Australia.

Inman, A. G., & DeBoer Kreider, E. (2013). Multicultural competence: Psychotherapy practice and supervision. *Psychotherapy, 50*(3), 346–350.

Insel, T. R., & Gogtay, N. (2014). National Institute of Mental Health clinical trials: New approaches, new expectations. *Journal of the American Medical Association Psychiatry, 71*(7), 745–746.

Jacobs, D., David, P., & Meyer, D. J. (1995). *The supervisory encounter: A guide for teachers of psychodynamic psychotherapy and analysis.* New Haven, CT: Yale University Press.

Jaffe, L. (2000). Supervision as an intersubjective process: Hearing from candidates and supervisors. *Journal of the American Psychoanalytic Association, 48*(2), 561–570.

Jaffe, L. (2001). Countertransference, supervised analysis, and psychoanalytic training requirements. *Journal of the American Psychoanalytic Association, 49*(3), 831–853.

January, A. M., Meyerson, D. A., Reddy, L. F., Docherty, A. R., & Klonoff, E. A. (2014). Impressions of misconduct: Graduate students' perception of faculty ethical violations in scientist-practitioner clinical psychology programs. *Training and Education in Professional Psychology, 8*(4), 261–268.

Jones, R. (2004). The science and meaning of the self. *Journal of Analytic Psychology, 49*(2), 217–233.

Jung, C. G. (1921). *Psychological types.* London: Routledge & Kegan Paul.

Jurist, E. (2018). *Minding emotions: Cultivating mentalization in psychotherapy.* New York: Guilford Press.

Kairys, D. (1964). The training analysis: A critical review of the literature and a controversial proposal. *Psychoanalytic Quarterly, 33*(4), 485–512.

Kantrowitz, J. (2002). The triadic match: The interactive effect of supervisor, candidate and patient. *Journal of the American Psychoanalytic Association, 50*(3), 939–968.

Kardiner, A. (1977). *My analysis with Freud: Reminiscences.* New York: Norton.

Karon, B. (2002). Analyzability or the inability to analyze? *Contemporary Psychoanalysis, 28*(1), 121–140.

Kassan, L. D. (2010). *Peer supervision groups: How they work and why you need one.* Northvale, NJ: Jason Aronson.

Keefe, J. R., McCarthy, K. S., Dinger, U., Zilcha-Mano, S., & Barber, J. P. (2014). A meta-analytic review of psychodynamic therapies for anxiety disorders. *Clinical Psychology Review, 34*(4), 309–323.

Kernberg, O. F. (1975). *Borderline conditions and pathological narcissism.* New York: Jason Aronson.

Kernberg, O. F. (1984). *Severe personality disorders: Psychotherapeutic strategies.* New Haven, CT: Yale University Press.

Kernberg, O. F. (1986). Institutional problems in psychoanalytic education. *Journal of the American Psychoanalytic Association, 34*(4), 799–834.

Kernberg, O. F. (1988). Clinical dimensions of masochism. *Journal of the American Psychoanalytic Association, 36*(4), 1005–1029.

Kernberg, O. F. (1996). Thirty methods to destroy the creativity of psychoanalytic candidates. *International Journal of Psychoanalysis, 77*, 1031–1040.

Kernberg, O. F. (1998). *Ideology, conflict, and leadership in groups and organizations*. New Haven, CT: Yale University Press.

Kernberg, O. F. (2000). A concerned critique of psychoanalytic education. *International Journal of Psychoanalysis, 81*, 97–120.

Kernberg, O. F. (2010). Psychoanalytic supervision: The supervisor's tasks. *Psychoanalytic Quarterly, 79*(3), 603–627.

Kernberg, O. F. (2014a). An overview of the treatment of severe narcissistic pathology. *International Journal of Psychoanalysis, 95*(5), 865–888.

Kernberg, O. F. (2014b). The twilight of the training analysis system. *Psychoanalytic Review, 101*(2), 151–174.

Kernberg, O. F. (2016). *Psychoanalytic education at the crossroads: Reformation, change and the future of psychoanalytic training*. London: Routledge.

Kernberg, O. F., & Michels, R. (2016). Thoughts on the present and future of psychoanalytic education. *Journal of the American Psychoanalytic Association, 64*(3), 477–493.

Kets de Vries, M., & Miller, D. (1984). *The neurotic organization*. San Francisco: Jossey-Bass.

Killingmo, B., Varvin, S., & Strømme, H. (2014). What can we expect from trainee therapists? A study of acquisition of competence in dynamic psychotherapy. *Scandinavian Psychoanalytic Review, 37*(1), 24–35.

Kim, S., & Strathearn, L. (2017). Trauma, mothering, and intergenerational transmission: A synthesis of behavioral and oxytocin research. *Psychoanalytic Study of the Child, 70*, 200–223.

Kirsner, D. (2000). *Unfree associations: Inside psychoanalytic institutes*. London: Process Press.

Klein, M. (1946). Notes on some schizoid mechanisms. *International Journal of Psychoanalysis, 27*, 99–110.

Kohon, G. (1999). *The dead mother: The work of André Green*. London: Routledge.

Kohut, H. (1971). *The analysis of the self*. New York: International Universities Press.

Kohut, H. (1977). *The restoration of the self*. New York: International Universities Press.

Kovacs, V. (1936). Training and control analysis. *International Journal of Psychoanalysis, 17*, 346–354.

Krupnik, J. L., Sotsky, S. M., Elkin, I., Simmens, S., Moyer, J., Watkins, J., & Pilkonis, P. A. (2006). The role of the therapeutic alliance in psychotherapy and pharmacotherapy outcome: Findings in the National Institute of Mental Health Treatment of Depression Collaborative Research Program. *Focus, 4*(2), 269–277.

Ladany, N. (2007). Does psychotherapy training matter? Maybe not. *Psychotherapy: Theory, Research, Practice, Training, 44*(4), 392–396.

Ladany, N., Hill, C. E., Corbett, M. M., & Nutt, E. D. (1996). Nature, extent, and importance of what psychotherapy trainees do not disclose to their supervisors. *Journal of Counseling Psychology 43*(1), 10–24.

Lane, R. D., Weihs, K. L., Herring, A., Hishaw, A., & Smith, R. (2015). Affective agnosia: Expansion of the alexithymia construct and a new opportunity to integrate and extend Freud's legacy. *Neuroscience and Behavioral Reviews,* 55(Aug.), 594–611.

Lasch, C. (1978). *Culture of narcissism: American life in an age of diminishing expectations.* New York: Norton.

Lauro, L., Bass, A., Goldsmith, S. A., Kaplan, J. A., Katz, G., & Shaye, S. H. (2003). Psychoanalytic supervision of the difficult patient. *Psychoanalytic Quarterly,* 72(2), 403–437.

Layton, L. (2016). Commentary on Kernberg and Michels. *Journal of the American Psychoanalytic Association,* 64(3), 501–510.

Layton, L., Hollander, N. C., & Gutwill, S. (Eds.). (2006). *Psychoanalysis, class, and politics: Encounters in the clinical setting.* New York: Routledge.

Layton, L., & Leavy-Sperounis, M. (2020). *Toward a social psychoanalysis: Culture, character, and normative unconscious processes.* New York: Routledge.

Leamy, M., Bird, V., Le Boutillier, C., & Williams, J. (2011). Conceptual framework for personal recovery in mental health: Systematic review and narrative syntheses. *British Journal of Psychiatry,* 199(6), 445–452.

Leary, K. (2000). Racial enactments in dynamic treatment. *Psychoanalytic Dialogues,* 10(4), 639–653.

Lehrman-Waterman, D., & Ladany, N. (2001). Development and validation of the evaluation process within supervision inventory. *Journal of Counseling Psychology,* 48(2), 168–177.

Leichsenring, F., Luyten, P., Hilsenroth, M. J., Abbass, A., & Barber, J. P. (2015). Psychodynamic therapy meets evidence-based medicine: A systematic review using updated criteria. *Lancet Psychiatry,* 2(7), 648–660.

Lemma, A. (2018). Transitory identities: Some psychoanalytic reflections on transgender identities. *International Journal of Psychoanalysis,* 99(5), 1089–1106.

Levendosky, A. A., & Hopwood, C. J. (2016). A clinical science approach to training first year clinicians to navigate therapeutic relationships. *Journal of Psychotherapy Integration,* 27(2), 153–171.

Levenson, E. A. (1982). Follow the fox—An inquiry into the vicissitudes of psychoanalytic supervision. *Contemporary Psychoanalysis,* 18(1), 1–15.

Levenson, E. A. (1988). The pursuit of the particular. *Contemporary Psychoanalysis,* 24(1), 1–16.

Levine, P., & Frederick, A. (1997). *Waking the tiger: Healing trauma.* Berkeley, CA: North Atlantic Books.

Levy, S. T. (2016). Commentary on Kernberg and Michels. *Journal of the American Psychoanalytic Association,* 64(3), 511–515.

Lifschutz, J. E. (1976). A critique of reporting and assessment in the training analysis. *Journal of the American Psychoanalytic Association,* 24(1), 43–59.

Linehan, M. M. (1993). *Cognitive-behavioral treatment of borderline personality disorder.* New York: Guilford Press.

Lingiardi, V., & Capozzi, P. (2004). Psychoanalytic attitudes toward homosexuality. *International Journal of Psychoanalysis,* 85(1), 137–158.

Lingiardi, V., & McWilliams, N. (Eds.). (2017). *Psychodynamic diagnostic manual (PDM-2)* (2nd ed.). New York: Guilford Press.

Lingiardi, V., McWilliams, N., & Muzi, L. (2017). The contributions of Sidney Blatt's two-polarities model to the *Psychodynamic Diagnostic Manual. Research in Psychotherapy: Process and Outcome,* 20(1), 12–18.

Lopez, S. J., Pedrotti, J. T., & Snyder, C. R. (2018). *Positive psychology: The science and practical exploration of human strengths* (4th ed.). New York: Sage.

Luyten, P., Vliegen, N., Van Houdenhove, B., & Blatt, S. J. (2008). Equifinality, multifinality, and the rediscovery of the importance of early experiences. *Psychoanalytic Study of the Child, 63,* 27–60.

Mammen, M. A. (2020). Attachment dynamics in the supervisory relationship: Becoming your own good supervisor. *Journal of Psychotherapy Integration, 30*(1), 93–101.

Maroda, K. J. (1991). *The power of countertransference.* Northvale, NJ: Aronson.

Maroda, K. J. (1999). *Seduction, surrender, and transformation: Emotional engagement in the analytic process.* Hillsdale, NJ: Analytic Press.

Martindale, B., Mörner, M., Cid Rodriguez, M. E., & Vidit, J.-P. (Eds.). (1997). *Supervision and its vicissitudes.* London: Karnac.

Maslow, A. H. (1943). A theory of human motivation. *Psychological Review, 50*(4), 370–396.

McDougall, J. (1980). *Plea for a measure of abnormality.* New York: International Universities Press.

McRuer, R. (2006). Compulsory able-bodiedness and queer/disabled existence. In L. J. Davis (Ed.), *The disability studies reader* (4th ed., pp. 369–378). New York: Routledge.

McWilliams, N. (1987). The grandiose self and the interminable analysis. *Current Issues in Psychoanalytic Practice, 4*(3–4), 93–107.

McWilliams, N. (2003). The educative aspects of psychoanalysis. *Psychoanalytic Psychology, 20*(2), 245-260.

McWilliams, N. (2004). *Psychoanalytic psychotherapy: A practitioner's guide.* New York: Guilford Press.

McWilliams, N. (2005). Preserving our humanity as therapists. *Psychotherapy: Theory, Research, Practice, Training, 24*(2), 139–151.

McWilliams, N. (2006). Some thoughts about schizoid dynamics. *Psychoanalytic Review, 93*(1), 1–24.

McWilliams, N. (2011). *Psychoanalytic diagnosis: Understanding personality structure in the clinical* process (2nd ed.). New York: Guilford Press.

McWilliams, N. (2016). Commentary on Kernberg and Michels. *Journal of the American Psychoanalytic Association, 64*(3), 517–524.

McWilliams, N. (2019). The future of psychoanalysis: Preserving Jeremy Safran's integrative vision. *Psychoanalytic Psychology, 37*(2), 98–107.

McWilliams, N., & Stein, J. (1987). Women's groups run by women: The management of devaluing transferences. *International Journal of Group Psychotherapy, 37*(2), 139–153.

Meares, R. (2012a). *Borderline personality disorder and the conversational model: A clinician's manual.* New York: Norton.

Meares, R. (2012b). *A dissociation model of borderline personality disorder.* New York: Norton.

Mehr, K. E., Ladany, N., & Caskie, G. I. L. (2015). Factors influencing trainee willingness to disclose in supervision. *Training and Education in Professional Psychology, 9*(1), 44–51.

Meissner, W. W. (1978). *The paranoid process.* New York: Jason Aronson.

Meloy. J. R. (1988). *The psychopathic mind: Origins, dynamics, and treatment.* Northvale, NJ: Jason Aronson.

Menzies, I. E. P. (1960). A case-study in the functioning of social systems as a defence against anxiety: A report on a study of the nursing service of a general hospital. *Human Relations, 13*(2), 95–121.

Mesrie, V., Diener, M. J., & Clark, A. (2018). Trainee attachment to supervisor and perceptions of novice psychotherapist counseling self-efficacy: The moderating role of level of experience. *Psychotherapy, 55*(3), 216–221.

Messer, S., & McWilliams, N. (2006). Insight in psychodynamic therapy. In L. Castonguay & C. Hill (Eds.), *Insight in psychotherapy* (pp. 9–29). New York: Springer.

Mikulincer, M., & Shaver, P. R. (2016). *Attachment in adulthood: Structure, dynamics, and change* (2nd ed.). New York: Guilford Press.

Miller, A. (1975). *Prisoners of childhood: The drama of the gifted child and the search for the true self.* New York: Basic Books.

Miller, L., & Twomey, J. E. (1999). A parallel without a process: A relational view of a supervisory experience. *Contemporary Psychoanalysis, 35*(4), 557–580.

Moga, D. E., & Cabaniss, D. W. (2014). Learning objectives for supervision: Benefits for candidates and beyond. *Psychoanalytic Inquiry, 34*(6), 528–537.

Mucci, C. (2013). *Beyond individual and collective trauma: Intergenerational transmission, psychoanalytic treatment, and the dynamics of forgiveness.* New York: Routledge.

Mucci, C. (2018). *Borderline bodies: Affect regulation for personality disorders.* New York: Norton.

Mulay, A. L., Kelly, E., & Cain, N. (2017). Psychodynamic treatment of the criminal offender: Making the case for long-term treatment in a longer-term setting. *Psychodynamic Psychiatry, 45*(2), 143–173.

Nagell, W., Steinmetzer, L., Fissabre, U., & Spilski, J. (2014). Research into the relationship experience in supervision and its influence on the psychoanalytic identity formation of candidate trainees. *Psychoanalytic Inquiry, 34*(6), 554–583.

Norcross, J. C., & Wampold, B. E. (2011). Evidence-based therapy relationships: Conclusions and clinical practices. *Psychotherapy, 48*(1), 98–102.

Norcross, J. C., & Wampold, B. E. (2019). Relationships and responsiveness in the psychological treatment of trauma: The tragedy of the APA clinical practice guidelines. *Psychotherapy: Theory, Research, Practice, Training, 56*(3), 391–399.

O'Donovan, A., & Kavanagh, D. J. (2014). Measuring competence in supervisees and supervisors: Satisfaction and related reactions in supervision. In C. E. Watkins, Jr. & D. L. Miller. (Eds.), *The Wiley international handbook of clinical supervision* (pp. 458–467). New York: Wiley.

Ogden, P., Pain, C., & Minton, K. (2006). *Trauma and the body: A sensorimotor approach to psychotherapy.* New York: Norton.

Ogden, T. H. (2005). On psychoanalytic supervision. *International Journal of Psychoanalysis, 86*(5), 1265–1280.

Oldham, J. M., & Bone, S. (1997). *Paranoia: New psychoanalytic perspectives.* Madison, CT: International Universities Press.

Panizza, S. (2014). Vitality: Its thousand faces. *The Italian Psychoanalytic Annual, 8*, 25–39.

Panksepp, J. (1998). *Affective neuroscience. The foundations of human and animal emotions.* New York: Oxford University Press.

Panksepp, J., & Biven, L. (2012). *The archeology of mind: Neuroevolutionary origins of human emotions.* New York: Norton.

PDM Task Force. (2006). *Psychodynamic diagnostic manual.* Silver Spring, MD: Alliance of Psychoanalytic Organizations.

Pearlman, L.A., & Saakvitne, K. (1995). *Trauma and the therapist: Countertransference and vicarious traumatization in psychotherapy with incest survivors.* New York: Norton.

Peebles-Kleiger, M. J., Horwitz, L., Kleiger, J. H., & Waugaman, R. M. (2006). Psychological testing and analyzability: Breathing new life into an old issue. *Psychoanalytic Psychology, 23*(3), 504–526.

Perlman, S. D. (1996). The implications of transference and parallel process for the frame of supervision. *Journal of the American Academy of Dynamic Psychiatry, 24*(3), 485–497.

Petts, A., & Shapley, B. (Eds.). (2007). *On supervision: Psychoanalytic and Jungian perspectives.* London: Karnac.

Piaget, J. (2011). *The language and thought of the child.* New York: Routledge. (Original work published 1923)

Pieterse, A. L. (2018). Attending to racial trauma in clinical supervision: Enhancing client and supervisee outcomes. *The Clinical Supervisor, 37*(1), 204–220.

Pine, F. (2020). On observation, theory, and the mind of the working clinician. *Psychoanalytic Psychology, 37*(2), 89–97.

Pizer, B. (1997). When the analyst is ill: Dimensions of self-disclosure. *Psychoanalytic Quarterly, 66*(3), 450–469.

Plakun, E. M., Sudak, D. M., & Goldberg, D. (2009). The Y model: An integrated, evidence-based approach to teaching psychotherapy competencies. *Journal of Psychiatric Practice, 15*(1), 5–11.

Power, A. (2009). Supervision—A space where diversity can be thought about? *Attachment: New directions in psychotherapy and relational psychoanalysis, 3*(2), 157–175.

Rachman, A. W. (Ed.). (2016). *The Budapest school of psychoanalysis: The origin of a two-person psychology and empathic perspective.* New York: Routledge.

Racker, H. (1968). *Transference and countertransference.* New York: International Universities Press.

Rangell, L. (1982). Transference to theory: The relationship of psychoanalytic education to the analyst's relationship to psychoanalysis. *Annual of Psychoanalysis, 10*(1), 29–56.

Reeder, J. (2004). *Hate and love in psychoanalytic institutions: Dilemmas of a profession.* New York: Other Press.

Reik, T. (1948). *Listening with the third ear: The inner experience of a psychoanalyst.* New York: Farrar, Straus.

Rice, A. K. (1965). *Learning for leadership.* London: Tavistock.

Rice, A. K. (1969). Individual, group, and intergroup processes. *Human Relations, 22*(6), 565–584.

Richardson, J., Cabaniss, D. L., Halperin, J., Vaughan, S. C., & Cherry, S. (2020). Beyond progression: Devising a new training model for candidate assessment, advancement, and advising at Columbia. *Journal of the American Psychoanalytic Association, 68*(2), 201–216.

Robbins, A. (1988). *Between therapists: The processing of transference/countertransference material.* New York: Human Sciences Press.

Robbins, A. (2020). The elderly therapist/patient: The developmental challenge of expansion and contraction and other reflections of an aging psychoanalyst. *Psychoanalytic Review, 107*(5), 395–404.

Rock, M. H. (Ed.). (1997). *Psychodynamic supervision: Perspectives of the supervisor and the supervisee.* Northvale, NJ: Jason Aronson.

Rosbrow, T. (1997). From parallel process to developmental process: A developmental/plan formulation approach to supervision. In M. H. Rock (Ed.). *Psychodynamic supervision: Perspectives of the supervisor and the supervisee* (pp. 213–236). Northvale, NJ: Jason Aronson.

Rousmaniere, T. (2016). *Deliberate practice for psychotherapists: A guide to improving clinical effectiveness.* New York: Routledge.

Roustang, F. (1982). *Dire mastery: From Freud to Lacan.* Baltimore: Johns Hopkins University Press.

Ryan, J. (2018). *Class and psychoanalysis: Landscapes of inequality.* London: Routledge.

Safran, J. D., & Muran, J. C. (2003). *Negotiating the therapeutic alliance: A relational treatment guide.* New York: Guilford Press.

Saketopoulou, A. (2011). Minding the gap: Intersections between gender, race, and class in work with gender variant children. *Psychoanalytic Dialogues, 21*(2), 192–209.

Sarnat, J. (2010). Key competencies of the psychodynamic psychotherapist and how to teach them in supervision. *Psychotherapy: Theory, Research, Practice, Training, 47*(1), 20–27.

Sarnat, J. (2015). *Supervision essentials for psychodynamic psychotherapies.* Washington, DC: American Psychological Association.

Sarnat, J. (2019). What's new in parallel process? The evolution of supervision's signature phenomenon. *American Journal of Psychoanalysis, 79*(3), 304–328.

Schafer, R. (1968). *Aspects of internalization.* New York: International Universities Press.

Schafer, R. (1979). On becoming a psychoanalyst of one persuasion or another. *Contemporary Psychoanalysis, 15*(3), 345–360.

Schafer, R. (1983). *The analytic attitude.* New York: Basic Books.

Scharff, J. S. (Ed.). (2018). *Clinical supervision of psychoanalytic psychotherapy.* New York: Routledge.

Schein, E. (1985). *Organizational culture and leadership.* San Francisco: Jossey-Bass.

Schen, C. R., & Greenlee, A. (2018). Race in supervision: Let's talk about it. *Psychodynamic Psychiatry, 46*(1), 1–21.

Schore, A. N. (2016). The right brain implicit self: A central mechanism of the psychotherapy change process. In G. Craparo & C. Mucci (Eds.), *Unrepressed unconscious, implicit memory, and clinical work* (pp. 73–98). London: Karnac.

Schore, A. N. (2019). *Right brain psychotherapy.* New York: Norton.

Searles, H. (1955). The informational value of the supervisor's emotional experience. *Psychiatry, 18*(2), 135–146.

Searles, H. (1962). Problems of psycho-analytic supervision. In *Collected papers on schizophrenia and related subjects* (pp. 584–604). New York: International Universities Press.

Seinfeld, J. (1991). *The empty core: An object relations approach to psychotherapy of the schizoid personality.* Northvale, NJ: Jason Aronson.

Seligman, M. E. P. (1995). The effectiveness of psychotherapy: The *Consumer Reports* study. *American Psychologist, 50*(12), 965–974.

Seligman, M. E. P. (2004). *Authentic happiness: Using the new positive psychology to realize your potential for lasting fulfillment.* New York: Atria Books.

Seligman, S. (2016). Commentary on Kernberg and Michels. *Journal of the American Psychoanalytic Association, 64*(3), 525–533.

Shapiro, D. (1965). *Neurotic styles.* New York: Basic Books.

Shapiro, F., & Forrest, M. S. (Eds.). (1997). *EMDR, the breakthrough "eye movement" therapy for overcoming anxiety, stress and trauma.* New York: Basic Books.

Sharp, C., Wright, A. G. C., Fowler, J. C., Frueh, B. C., Allen, J. G., Oldham, J., & Clark, L. A. (2015). The structure of personality pathology: Both general ('g') and specific ('s') factors? *Journal of Abnormal Psychology, 124*(2), 387–398.

Shedler, J. (2010). The efficacy of psychodynamic psychotherapy. *American Psychologist, 65*(2), 98–109.

Shedler, J. (2015). Integrating clinical and empirical perspectives on personality: The Shedler–Westen Assessment Procedure (SWAP). In S. K. Huprich (Ed.), *Personality disorders: Toward theoretical and empirical integration in diagnosis and treatment* (pp. 225–252). Washington, DC: American Psychological Association.

Shedler, J. (2019). A psychiatric diagnosis is not a disease: Doublethink makes for bad treatment. Retrieved from *psychologytoday.com/us/blog/psychologically-minded/201907/psychiatric-illness-is-not-a-disease.*

Shedler, J., & Aftab, A. (2020, July 29). Psychoanalysis and the re-enchantment of psychiatry: Jonathan Shedler, PhD. *Psychiatric Times.* Retrieved from *www.psychiatrictimes.com/view/psychoanalysis-re-enchantment-psychiatry-jonathan-shedler-phd.*

Shedler, J., & Westen, D. (2004). Refining personality disorder diagnosis: Integrating science and practice. *American Journal of Psychiatry, 161*(8), 1350–1365.

Shengold, L. (1989). *Soul murder: The effects of childhood abuse and deprivation.* New Haven, CT: Yale University Press.

Sherman, E. (2015). Mutual anxiety in supervision. *Psychoanalytic Perspectives, 12*(2), 179—191.

Shevrin, H. (1981). On being the analyst supervised. In R. Wallerstein (Ed.), *Becoming a psychoanalyst: A study of psychoanalytic supervision* (pp. 322–325). New York: International Universities Press.

Siassi, S. (2013). *Forgiveness in intimate relationships: A psychoanalytic perspective.* London: Karnac.

Sifneos, P. (1973). The prevalence of "alexithymia" characteristics in psychosomatic patients. *Psychotherapy and Psychosomatics, 22,* 255–262.

Silberschatz, G. (2005). *Transformative relationships: The control-mastery theory of psychotherapy.* New York: Routledge.

Slavin, J. (1998). Influence and vulnerability in psychoanalytic supervision and treatment. *Psychoanalytic Psychology, 15*(2), 230–244.

Sloane, P. (1957). The technique of supervised analysis. *Journal of the American Psychoanalytic Association, 5*(2), 539–547.

Smith, K. R. (2021a). *The ethical visions of psychotherapy.* New York: Routledge.

Smith, K. R. (2021b). *Therapeutic ethics in context and in dialogue.* New York: Routledge.

Solomon, A. (2012). *Far from the tree: Parents, children, and the search for identity.* New York: Scribner.

Solye, K., & Strathearn, L. (2017). Trauma, mothering, and intergenerational transmission: A synthesis of behavioral and oxytocin research. *Psychoanalytic Study of the Child, 70,* 200–223.

Soreanu, R. (2019). Supervision for our times: Countertransference and the rich legacy of the Budapest School. *American Journal of Psychoanalysis, 79*(3), 329–351.

Steinert, C., Munder, T., Rabung, S., Hoyer, J., & Leichsenring, F. (2017). Psychodynamic therapy: As efficacious as other empirically supported treatments? A meta-analysis testing equivalence of outcomes. *American Journal of Psychiatry, 174*(10) 943–953.

Sterba, R. (1934). The fate of the ego in analytic therapy. *International Journal of Psychoanalysis, 15,* 117–126.

Stern, D. B. (1997). *Unformulated experience: From dissociation to imagination in psychoanalysis.* Hillsdale, NJ: Analytic Press.

Stern, D. B. (2009). *Partners in thought: Working with unformulated experience, dissociation, and enactment.* New York: Routledge.

Sternberg, R. J. (2003). *Wisdom, intelligence, and creativity synthesized.* New York: Cambridge University Press.

Strømme, H. (2012). Confronting helplessness: A study of the acquisition of dynamic psychotherapeutic competence by psychology students. *Nordic Psychology, 64*(3), 203–217.

Strømme, H. (2014). A bad and better supervision process; actualized relational scenarios in trainees: A longitudinal study of nondisclosure in psychodynamic supervision. *Psychoanalytic Inquiry, 34*(6), 584–605.

Strømme, H., & Gullestad, S. E. (2012). Disclosure or non-disclosure? An in-depth study of psychodynamic supervision. *Scandinavian Psychoanalytic Review, 35*(2), 105–115.

Strupp, H., Hadley, S., & Gomez-Schwartz, B. (1977). *Psychotherapy for better or worse: An analysis of the problem of negative effects.* New York: Jason Aronson.

Suchet, M. (2007). Unraveling whiteness. *Psychoanalytic Dialogues, 17*(6), 867–886.

Sue, D. W. (2010). *Microaggressions in everyday life: Race, gender, and sexual orientation.* Hoboken, NJ: Wiley.

Sullivan, H. S. (1953). *The interpersonal theory of psychiatry.* New York: Norton.

Sulloway, F. J. (1996). *Born to rebel: Birth order, family dynamics, and creative lives.* New York: Pantheon.

Szecsödy, I. (1989). Supervision: A didactic or mutative situation. *Psychoanalytic Psychotherapy 4*(3), 245–261.

Szecsödy, I. (2008). Does anything go in psychoanalytic supervision? *Psychoanalytic Inquiry, 28*(3), 373–386.

Szecsody, I. (2013). *Supervision and the making of the psychoanalyst*. Washington, DC: International Psychotherapy Institute Books.

Tarasoff v. Board of Regents of the University of California, 17 Cal. 3rd 425 (Cal. 1976).

Taylor, G. J., & Bagby, R. M. (2013). Psychoanalysis and empirical research: The example of alexithymia. *Journal of the American Psychoanalytic Association, 61*(1), 99–133.

Teitelman, S. (1995). The changing scene in psychoanalytic supervision. *Psychoanalysis and Psychotherapy, 12*(2), 183–192.

Thompson, M. G. (2004). *The ethic of honesty: The fundamental rule of psychoanalysis*. New York: Rodopi.

Ticho, E.A. (1972). Termination of psychoanalysis: Treatment goals, life goals. *Psychoanalytic Quarterly, 41*(3), 315–333.

Tracey, T. J. G., Bludworth, J., & Glidden-Tracey, C. E. (2012). Are there parallel processes in psychotherapy supervision?: An empirical examination. *Psychotherapy, 49*(2), 330–343.

Tummala-Narra, P. (2004). Dynamics of race and culture in the supervisory encounter. *Psychoanalytic Psychology, 21*(2), 300–311.

Tummala-Narra, P. (2009). Teaching on diversity. *Psychoanalytic Psychology, 26*(3), 322–334.

Tummala-Narra, P. (2016). *Psychoanalytic theory and cultural competence in psychotherapy*. Washington, DC: American Psychological Association.

Vaughan, S. C., Spitzer, R., Davies, M., & Roose, S. P. (1997). The definition and assessment of analytic process: Can analysts agree? *International Journal of Psychoanalysis, 78*, 959–973.

Vivona, J. M. (2013). Psychoanalysis as poetry. *Journal of the American Psychoanalytic Association, 61*(6), 1109–1137.

Vollmer, G., & Bernardi, R. (1996). The multiple functions of the supervisor: A summary of the seventh IPA conference of training analysis. *International Journal of Psychoanalysis, 77*, 813–818.

Waelder, R. (1936). The principle of multiple function: Observations on over-determination. *Psychoanalytic Quarterly, 5*(1), 45–62.

Walker, M. (2004). Supervising practitioners working with survivors of childhood abuse: Countertransference, secondary traumatization and terror. *Psychodynamic Practice: Individuals, Groups and Organisations, 10*(2), 173–193.

Wallerstein, R. S. (1981). *Becoming a psychoanalyst*. New York: International Universities Press.

Wallerstein, R. S. (Ed.). (1992). *The common ground of psychoanalysis*. Northvale, NJ: Jason Aronson.

Wallerstein, R. S. (2010). The training analysis: Psychoanalysis's perpetual problem. *Psychoanalytic Review, 97*(6), 903–936.

Washton, A. M., & Zweben, J. E. (2006). *Treating alcohol and drug problems in psychotherapy practice: Doing what works*. New York: Guilford Press.

Watkins, C. E., Jr. (2011). Celebrating psychoanalytic supervision: Considering a century of seminal contribution. *Psychoanalytic Review, 98*(3), 401–418.

Watkins, C. E., Jr. (2013a). The beginnings of psychoanalytic supervision: The crucial role of Max Eitingon. *American Journal of Psychoanalysis, 73*(3), 254–270.

Watkins, C. E., Jr. (2013b). On psychoanalytic supervisor competencies, the persistent paradox without parallel in psychoanalytic education, and dreaming of an evidence-based psychoanalytic supervision. *Psychoanalytic Review, 100*(4), 609–646.

Watkins, C. E., Jr. (2015a). The evolving nature of psychoanalytic supervision: From pedagogical to andragogical perspective. *International Forum of Psychoanalysis, 24*(4), 230–242.

Watkins, C. E., Jr. (2015b). The learning alliance in psychoanalytic supervision: A fifty-year retrospective and prospective. *Psychoanalytic Psychology, 32*(3), 451–481.

Watkins, C. E., Jr. (2015c). Toward a research-informed, evidence-based psychoanalytic supervision. *Psychoanalytic Psychotherapy, 29*(1), 5–19.

Watkins, C. E., Jr. (2016). Listening to and sharing of self in psychoanalytic supervision: The supervisor's self-perspective. *Psychoanalytic Review, 103*(4), 565–579.

Watkins, C. E., Jr. (2017). Reconsidering parallel process in psychotherapy supervision: On parsimony, rival hypotheses, and alternative explanations. *Psychoanalytic Psychology, 34*(4), 506–515.

Watkins, C. E., Jr., & Hook, J. N. (2016). On a culturally humble psychoanalytic supervision perspective: Creating the cultural third. *Psychoanalytic Psychology, 33*(3), 487–517.

Watkins, C. E., Jr., Hook, J. N., Owen, J., DeBlaere, C., Davis, D. E., & Callahan, J. L. (2019). Creating and elaborating the cultural third: A doers-doing with perspective on psychoanalytic supervision. *American Journal of Psychoanalysis, 79*(3), 352–374.

Watkins, C. E., Jr., & Milne, D. L. (Eds.). (2014). *The Wiley international handbook of clinical supervision*. West Sussex, UK: Wiley Blackwell.

Watson, P., Raju, P., & Soklaridis, S. (2017). Teaching not-knowing: Strategies for cultural competence in psychotherapy supervision. *Academic Psychiatry, 41*(1), 55–61.

Weinberger, J., & Stoycheva, V. (2020). *The unconscious: Theory, research, and clinical implications*. New York: Guilford Press.

Weiner, J., Mizen, R., & Duckham, J. (Eds.). (2003). *Supervising and being supervised: A practice in search of a theory*. New York: Palgrave Macmillan.

Weiss, J. (1993). *How psychotherapy works: Process and technique*. New York: Guilford Press.

Westen, D. (1998). The scientific legacy of Sigmund Freud: Toward a psychodynamically informed psychological science. *Psychological Bulletin, 124*(3), 333–371.

Westen, D. (2002). The language of psychoanalytic discourse. *Psychoanalytic Dialogues, 12*(6), 857–898.

Wheelis, A. (1956). The vocational hazards of psychoanalysis. *International Journal of Psychoanalysis, 37*, 171–184.

Wilner, W. (2015). The interpenetration of supervision and psychotherapy. *Psychoanalytic Perspectives, 12*(2), 192–199.

Winnicott, D. W. (1953). Transitional objects and transitional phenomena. *International Journal of Psychoanalysis, 34,* 89–97.

Winnicott, D. W. (1960). Ego distortion in relation to the real and false self. In *The maturational process and the facilitating environment* (pp. 140–152). New York: International Universities Press.

Winnicott, D. W. (1963). From dependence towards independence in the development of the individual. In *The maturational process and the facilitating environment* (pp. 83–92). New York: International Universities Press, 1965.

Winnicott, D. W. (1965). *The maturational process and the facilitating environment.* New York: International Universities Press.

Winnicott, D. W. (1968). The use of an object. *International Journal of Psychoanalysis, 50,* 711–716.

Winnicott, D. W. (1971), *Therapeutic consultations in child psychiatry.* London: Hogarth Press.

Winograd, B. (Director). (2014). *Black psychoanalysts speak.* PEP Video Grants.

Wolf, E. S. (1988). *Treating the self: Elements of clinical self psychology.* New York: Guilford Press.

Wrape, E. R., Callahan J. L., Rieck, T., & Watkins, C. E., Jr. (2017). Attachment theory within clinical supervision: Application of the conceptual to the empirical. *Psychoanalytic Psychotherapy, 31*(1), 37–54.

Yerushalmi, H. (2014). On regression and supervision. *International Forum of Psychoanalysis, 23*(4), 229–237.

Yerushalmi, H. (2018). Supervisees' unique experiential knowledge. *British Journal of Psychotherapy, 34*(1), 78–94.

Young-Bruehl, E. (2007). A brief history of prejudice studies. In H. Parens, A. Mahfouz, S. W. Twemlow, & D. E. Scharff (Eds.), *The future of prejudice: Psychoanalysis and the prevention of prejudice* (pp. 219–235). New York: Rowman & Littlefield.

Yourman, D. B., & Farber, B. A. (1996). Nondisclosure and distortion in psychotherapy supervision. *Psychotherapy: Theory, Research, Practice, Training, 33*(4), 567–575.

Zicht, S. R. (2019). Observations on the centrality of security in psychoanalytic supervision: A view from the interpersonal tradition and attachment perspective. *American Journal of Psychoanalysis, 79*(3), 375–387.

Author Index